Confused, Angry, Anxious?

of related interest

No Fighting, No Biting, No Screaming
How to Make Behaving Positively Possible for People with
Autism and Other Developmental Disabilities
Bo Hejlskov Elvén
ISBN 978 1 84905 126 2
eISBN 978 0 85700 322 5

Sulky, Rowdy, Rude?
Why kids really act out and what to do about it
Bo Hejlskov Elvén and Tina Wiman
ISBN 978 1 78592 213 8
eISBN 978 1 78450 492 2

Disruptive, Stubborn, Out of Control?
Why kids get confrontational in the classroom, and what to do about it
Bo Hejlskov Elvén
ISBN 978 1 78592 212 1
eISBN 978 1 78450 490 8

Frightened, Disturbed, Dangerous?
Why working with patients in psychiatric care can
be really difficult, and what to do about it
Bo Hejlskov Elvén and Sophie Abild McFarlane
ISBN 978 1 78592 214 5
eISBN 978 1 78450 493 9

Confused, Angry, Anxious?

Why working with older people in care really can be difficult, and what to do about it

Bo Hejlskov Elvén, Charlotte Agger and Iben Ljungmann

Jessica Kingsley *Publishers*
London and Philadelphia

First published in 2017
by Jessica Kingsley Publishers
73 Collier Street
London N1 9BE, UK
and
400 Market Street, Suite 400
Philadelphia, PA 19106, USA

www.jkp.com

Library of Congress Cataloging in Publication Data
A CIP catalog record for this book is available from the Library of Congress

British Library Cataloguing in Publication Data
A CIP catalogue record for this book is available from the British Library

ISBN: 978 1 78592 215 2
eISBN: 978 1 78450 494 6

Printed and bound in Great Britain

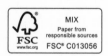

MIX
Paper from
responsible sources
FSC® C013056

Contents

Part 3: Extra Material

Introduction

It is difficult to prophesy. Especially about the future. But one thing we do know: Authorities around the world estimate that the number of people over 80 years old will increase by 45 per cent between 2020 and 2030. We know also that the older we become, the greater the risk of acquiring some form of dementia. Therefore it is a reasonable assumption that an ever-increasing number of people will be affected by dementia in the near future.

We also know that the number of beds in care homes for older people in most western countries has dwindled significantly in recent years. This development has brought about a dramatic change in the care of older people. Nowadays, residents at care homes suffer such significant physical and/ or mental disabilities that they are unable to manage day-to-day living on their own, in spite of maximal access to domiciliary care and community health services. As a result, residents at care homes need considerably more physical and mental care than in the past. At the same time, the complexity of their problems has increased greatly since older people, regardless of their health, are expected to be able to live in care homes. For example, mapping of the situation in Copenhagen municipality led to the estimate that 60–80 per cent of those who lived in normal care homes had dementia or dementia-like symptoms. This means that all those who work in care of older people must be able to cope with the behaviour that challenges and may arise as a result of dementia; it is part of the job. A part of the job that requires special skills.

At the same time, our attitude to those who need care has changed. Today the key words are right to self-determination and dignity. For this reason, care of older people today requires special knowledge and special skills. And, since we are able to supply specific competence in areas such as hygiene or wound-care, we should also be able to ensure that staff caring for older people have specific competence that enables them to understand and manage the types of behaviour that may occur in dementia illnesses.

When we authors have spoken to staff working in care of older people, they have told us of people with dementia with behaviour that challenges, for example refusing help with their personal hygiene, shouting, spitting, hitting and verbally abusing others. The staff then feel forced to resort to measures such as reprimands, sending the patient to his room, giving sedatives, or using physical intervention such as laying the person down on the floor, pushing them away in their wheelchair, or forcibly removing them from the scene. This naturally has the result that they experience feelings of powerlessness in such situations.

But while observing difficult care-giving situations such as these we have also seen that many older people, including those with dementia in older and dementia care, also seem helpless in the situation in which they find themselves. They express their desire not to have other people deciding for them and not to be subjected to what in patient-centred care is referred to as 'malignant' care. We will return to this topic later.

If those who are involved in caring for older people and for people with dementia do not change both their attitude and their understanding of this problem, then such care will become continuously more demanding and more expensive. This is why a book such as this is necessary.

Due to all the powerlessness we have come across in our work, both in care providers and many older people, we are always on the look-out for this feeling when training staff in older and dementia care. The reason is that we consider powerlessness itself to be absolutely the most devastating thing there is, regardless of whether it concerns staff or older people in a care home, or older people living with assistance in their own home.

It is easy to understand why powerlessness is devastating for older people. They are unable to influence their situation, they feel themselves to be in the power of either the staff or the illness, and life is experienced as just floating with the current. Their powerlessness increases as their abilities decline. From having been someone who managed perfectly well alone, perhaps raised children and participated in the community like everyone else, they have become dependent on others. Perhaps they even see before them how their dependency will continuously increase in the future.

But powerlessness is just as devastating for caregivers. Helpless staff often become confrontational and demanding. They may become cynical and resigned, and it may reach the point where they try to avoid the very people they are employed to care for. They prefer to sit in the office or staffroom rather than being present among older people who live in the home.

But worst of all is probably the powerlessness in the system itself, that shared impotence that is experienced by both staff and the older people. Instead of this being treated as a mutual problem, it rather serves to increase the opposition between the older people and caregivers. This can lead to an atmosphere of mutual distrust between the groups, with harsh speech and sometimes violence as the result. From older people with dementia in the form of hitting or kicking. From staff in the form of the use of force to get the older people into their rooms or, in the worst cases, use of physical restraint.

All involved may easily end up in situations such as these when their behaviours and methods don't work as expected. This is the very worst consequence of powerlessness.

INCREASED KNOWLEDGE AND EFFECTIVE, PROFESSIONAL HANDLING

The main purpose of this book is to give you who work in older and dementia care more knowledge about various types of behaviour that challenges, so that you can handle them effectively, professionally and with confidence. By learning to understand this type of behaviour and the methods described in the book, you and your colleagues will be able to change your shared everyday life in a positive direction.

Primarily it's all about looking at your own behaviour and the ways in which you handle difficult situations. Research has shown that changing your own behaviour is absolutely the most effective way to handle other people's behaviour.

THE MOST IMPORTANT GOAL OF
OLDER AND DEMENTIA CARE

The most important goal of older and dementia care is to ensure that the older people who need support in everyday life receive it, allowing them to live as full a life as possible. If they have dementia, however, the behaviour that challenges that may arise will make the task more difficult for the caregiver. To handle this as easily and smoothly as possible, caregivers should therefore concentrate on their primary function. The assignment then, is not to discipline people with dementia or to teach them to behave. Rather it is to manage and prevent their negative behaviours so that they can lead a functioning life. Preferably in a way that doesn't require too much time, energy or space. It is not the people with dementia whose task should be to behave themselves, rather it is the caregivers whose task it should be to create a context that allows these people's everyday life to function.

That's exactly what this book is about. How you who work in older and dementia care can think, act and interact with people with dementia, regardless of whether they live in a care home or in their own home. And how you can do this in a way that means you are taking responsibility to ensure that all older people with dementia can maintain a functioning life, with autonomy and the ability to take responsibility for their own actions.

TYPES OF DEMENTIA

Whenever you talk about dementia, it is important to point out that dementia is not expressed in the same way in all people. There are different types of dementia and they have different consequences for the affected person's behaviour. In a book such as this about behaviour that challenges, it is especially important to be aware of the types of dementia that exist and how they are expressed. For this reason, the Extra Material at the end of the book includes an overview of the four most common types of dementia: Alzheimer's disease, vascular dementia, frontotemporal dementia and Lewy Body dementia. Besides these four, there are many rarer forms of dementia, and it is not uncommon for a person to have more than one dementia illness at the same time.

The situations that you will read about in this book are real (anonymised), taken from daily life in various homes for people with dementia and for those who are just older. In the descriptions of each situation, we have deliberately not specified what type of dementia the people have. Our basic premise is that the approach chosen by the staff should not be based on the dementia diagnosis in itself. It should rather be a person-centred attitude that decides, in which each individual's resources and abilities, difficulties, interests, patterns of behaviour and ways of reacting are identified when the person is in various degrees of affect. To give you a general understanding of the different cognitive difficulties and symptoms that can be caused by the different types of dementia, so that you can recognise them in everyday life and understand why a certain person acts in the way they do, we recommend that you take a quick look at the different types of dementia in the Extra Material at the end of the book before reading any further. For example, it could be helpful to know that people with a certain type of dementia may suffer hallucinations, so that they will not be inappropriately treated with antipsychotic medication that has no effect on hallucinations in Lewy Body dementia.

Only by learning to understand the specific difficulties of an individual with dementia can one gain a feeling for what might work well in the next encounter with this person. For example, urinating in a flowerpot in the living room can be the result of different types of brain injury. It may be that due to frontal lobe damage the person doesn't care where he urinates. But it may also be that the person due to Alzheimer's disease misinterprets his surroundings and sees the flowerpot as a toilet or as a tree in the garden where he can relieve himself. Furthermore, a general understanding of the different types of dementia can give ideas for possible pedagogical solutions. For people with frontotemporal dementia, for example, you can very well calmly and clearly inform them where they should relieve themselves instead. With Alzheimer patients, however, you have to be very careful about pointing out faults and deficiencies, because they would actually feel quite ashamed. And of course you don't want anyone to feel ashamed. Because that's a fundamental principle of person-centred care.

PERSON-CENTRED CARE

Parallel to the shift in care for older people from providing care homes for the generally healthy and hospital care for the physically ill and older people with dementia, to older people's care of today where almost everyone receiving assistance has some kind of functional impairment, a way of thinking developed in the care of older people in Britain that is called 'person-centred care'. The main principles of this approach were developed by the British psychologist Tom Kitwood and have since been used and further developed around the world. They have even spread to other fields of care, such as obstetrics and general health care. Tom Kitwood's main point is that the person is more important than the diagnosis. You must first of all see the person, not the person's diagnosis.

This is a basically human thought; after all, we are all people, and should not be seen as objects of care. Tom Kitwood found that those who are treated as persons also behave as persons to a greater degree than if they are treated as objects of care. This means that the manner in which care of older people is delivered will have a significant effect on how a person with dementia is affected by his illness.

Kitwood describes how a standard of care, in which five fundamental psychological needs are addressed, enables a person with dementia to better handle their illness and to retain a higher level of functioning for a longer period of time. These five basic needs are:

1. *Comfort.* That the person with dementia receives comfort in the form of tenderness, closeness, soothing of anxiety and sorrow, reassurance, and the feeling of security that comes from having a fellow human being nearby. That staff keep things together when they are in danger of falling apart. When the person loses his self-control, the staff must not lose theirs, but rather help the person to regain control.

2. *Attachment.* That the person with dementia connects to others in such a way that he feels sure of being appreciated, regardless of his personal chaos. 'They still like me, even when I have a bad day.' That staff use the person's own perception of events as the point of departure, and acknowledge it.

3. *Inclusion.* That the person with dementia feels part of a fellowship and a greater context, where the feeling

is based on the assumption that the group would not manage as well if that person was not a part of it.

4. *Occupation.* That the person with dementia is engaged in meaningful activity that builds on his own abilities and life history, and that he is involved in both the process of life and routine activities.

5. *Identity.* That the person with dementia has a sense of identity, knows who he is, and can 'tell his own story'. The right to be seen and heard, and to be taken seriously.

But there is also care that is malignant and that hastens the progression of illness. Which often leads to behaviour that challenges. Tom Kitwood has identified 17 examples of this, and they are reviewed in detail in the Extra Material at the end of the book. These are examples in which the care is *not* founded on the patient's identity, resources and ability to act as an independent and social person.

To work in a person-centred way with people with dementia requires constant involvement. As caregiver, it's so easy to get stuck in a wish to educate or maybe even foster, even though education and fostering builds on learning and dementia actually means you're not very good at learning any more.

PERSON-CENTRED CARE AND THE LOW-AROUSAL APPROACH

The basic premise of this book is to create a link between person-centred care methods and the low-arousal approach (a method of managing behaviour that challenges that is best described by the principles that form the chapters of the book), since the two methods, or educational approaches, complement each other. It is easier to work in a person-centred way if you have practical methods for handling behaviour that challenges, and it is easier to work with the low-arousal approach if you are engaged in a person-centred culture of care.

We that have authored the book work in different ways with the low-arousal approach and with person-centred care. In Bo Hejlskov Elvén's work as a psychologist the low-arousal approach is central; and in Charlotte Agger's and Iben Ljungmann's work as leaders of a dementia centre, working in a person-centred way is central.

READING THIS BOOK

The purpose of this book is to create an openness that can settle accounts with ideas such as 'common sense' and 'personal chemistry' (expressions most of us use when we can't find arguments for why we do what we actually do) and instead lead you who work with older people, and especially those with dementia, to try to think and act in a different, more considerate, more respectful, and more effective way. But it will take both flexibility and openness.

The first part of the book is divided into 11 chapters, each dealing with a principle that is exemplified by at least one real-life situation. The principles are founded on research specifically relating to behaviour that challenges. Some of them are a far cry from how we normally think. But since you have chosen to read this book, it is probably because the principles you usually depend on have proved to be inadequate. We also discuss the situations and actions of the staff in the light of the different principles.

The second part consists of case studies of real-life interactions between older people and staff, and here we will look a little more broadly at the different situations against the background of the principles described in the first part. This can aid in understanding what is really happening and based on this possible strategies can then be formulated. The idea is to give you as a caregiver practical methods and an overall approach that you can use in your everyday work in homes for older people and for people with dementia. Because we are convinced that you often come across situations like those we describe.

In this book, where we could have written 'he or she', we have chosen to write 'he'. This is for practical purposes, to make the text easier to read. We also use the term 'older people', even though in most cases we are referring to people with dementia regardless of their age. This is also to make reading easier. And instead of filling the book with footnotes, we have chosen to collect in one place the reference texts that describe the research and theories presented in the book, chapter by chapter. This, too, is for increased readability. You will find the reference texts in the Study Materials at the end of the book. There you will also find study materials for each principle, which you can use as the basis for group discussions in your work team. The study materials consist of 12 group discussions. Each discussion is expected to take a quarter to half an hour, and they would fit well as the concluding business of a weekly staff meeting or the like.

Part 1

Principles

1

Always Identify the One With the Problem

DORA

Dora arrives in respite care in the middle of April. She roams around uneasily, and keeps coming in to the office to ask for her keys, since she wants to go home to her apartment. Today again, Dora wants her keys. She insists, saying in a very threatening way to Lisa who is in the office: 'I want my keys, and if you don't give them to me I'm going to the police; I know you're hiding them!' Then she starts rooting around in boxes and cabinets. When Lisa asks her to stop, she goes away. A little later, Lisa sees Dora crossing the road outside. She's on her way home.

PROBLEMS AND SOLUTIONS

The principle 'Always identify the one with the problem' is simple. In the example about Dora, a difficult situation ends with her leaving. For the staff, this is a big problem. For Dora it's a solution. Her incentive to change her behaviour is minimal. She solves a difficult problem in a way that seems excellent to her. But the staff have a dilemma. It is a huge problem to be responsible for someone who can't find their way, especially if that person wants to go back to their old home.

If the staff in this situation think that it is Dora who is behaving badly, then things will get difficult. Because then they will want her to change her behaviour. But Dora doesn't see it as a problem that she is leaving, and has no intention of changing her good solution for a worse one. Instead, Lisa and her colleagues have to ensure that the situation never gets this far. Their incentive to adjust their behaviour must be greater than Dora's is. They are the professionals. Dora is a resident in respite care. She has documented difficulties in coping with everyday life. In order to resolve the situation, first of all, here and now, a member of staff must go after Dora. As the next step, they must find a way to make sure that the same thing doesn't happen again. To keep Dora locked up in order to have better oversight of her is not a solution, nor is it logical or legal. Staff may not use force in order to gain better control.

Lisa goes after Dora. She doesn't run, but rather walks behind her calmly and quietly until she has caught up. Lisa asks: 'What are you going to do when you get home?' 'I'm going home because it's warm there,' says Dora, at the same time rubbing her bare arms. Lisa says: 'Dora, are you cold? Wouldn't you like to put on a warm sweater? Come, let's go inside and find you a warm sweater.' They walk back together and find a sweater, which Dora puts on. Dora sits down in the lounge and smiles and waves at Lisa as she walks back to the office.

FREDERICK
Frederick comes stomping out of his room shouting: 'Fire, fire!' Some of the staff come running and establish that there is in

fact no fire anywhere. Dunja, a nursing aide, says to him: 'No, there's no fire. No fire and no smoke.' Frederick pushes her aside and hurries down the corridor, still shouting: 'Fire, Fire!'

Dunja and some of her colleagues follow after Frederick and try to get him to stop, but he hits out at them and keeps on shouting, even louder than before. When they ask him to be quiet, he exerts himself still more. The staff call for the nurse and tell her that Frederick is completely paranoid and needs a sedative. The nurse goes up to Frederick and asks him: 'Where is the fire?' Frederick stops shouting and says: 'In the leg, in the leg.' The nurse replies: 'Does your leg hurt? Do you want something for the pain?' Frederick sits down obviously relieved and says: 'Yes please, and good thing you came along.'

In Frederick's case too, there is a reason for his behaviour. He has a sore leg but does not understand this. His interpretation, that something is burning, is a result of the difficulty he has in placing the pain in context. Since he thinks that something is on fire, it makes sense for him to run for help.

Dunja and the other members of staff don't understand what's going on. First, they try to correct Frederick's perception of reality (a fostering method with no respect for what he himself is perceiving) and, when that doesn't work, they come to the conclusion that he needs a sedative in order to calm down. Frederick's running and shouting is a problem for them. But for Frederick, it's a solution. His problem, of course, is that he is in pain. Only when the nurse asks what he is experiencing do the rest of the staff receive access to his problem, allowing it to be resolved. And thereby the staff's problem is also resolved. To expect Frederick to solve the staff's problem is not realistic – nor forward-thinking. That's why it doesn't help for them to ask Frederick to be quiet or to show him that there is no fire.

This book is about how we who work in caring for older people handle the problems we encounter. But from the very beginning, it must be pointed out that the problems we are discussing are the problems that we ourselves experience. In other words, the book is about how we can solve the problems we encounter, and not about what the older people can do to solve our problems. Most of the time, they solve their own problems. Perhaps not always using what we would consider the best methods, more often using methods that cause problems that have to be solved here and now. But as staff, we have to recognise that we have greater responsibility than those with whom we work – for several reasons. We are professionals. They are not. So it is natural that we should bear the responsibility. And only by accepting that responsibility can we solve the problems we encounter.

Summary
There is a tendency to look at behaviour that challenges as if it is the person exhibiting the behaviour that has the problem. In actual fact, problems arise when we don't know how to handle a certain kind of behaviour. In order to be effective we must therefore understand that when we lack methods for handling the behaviour, we are the ones with a problem.

2

People Behave Well
If They Can

ERIC

Eric keeps going to the fridge to get food. The staff consider this a big problem because Eric's hands are dirty when he's rooting through the food. They think this is inconsiderate of the health of the other residents. So they have repeatedly explained to Eric that he must not root around in the fridge, and they have tried to keep him in his room at mealtimes.

Today again, here comes Eric and wants to look in the fridge. Alice, a member of staff who happens to be in the kitchen, says: 'I can get food for you.' But Eric keeps going towards the fridge. Alice then places herself in front of the fridge to stop Eric from opening it: 'No, Eric, I have told you that you may not go into the fridge yourself.' He ignores Alice, takes hold of the door and pulls so that Alice falls over. Before she has a chance to move, he kicks her. Alice shouts: 'It is not OK for you to kick and hit people, do you hear me!' Then Eric pulls everything out of the fridge. Alice and the other people in the kitchen leave and lock themselves in one of the rooms. Eric carries on knocking over furniture and throwing it around the kitchen. After a little while, however, he goes off to his room.

Afterwards a meeting is held with the management, where the staff express their unanimous opinion that Eric does not belong in their department and that the management must have him moved. Otherwise, at the very least, there must be an extra member of staff available 24 hours a day for Eric, in order to protect the other residents at the home.

ABILITIES, REQUIREMENTS AND EXPECTATIONS

The principle 'People behave well if they can' was formulated by Ross W. Greene, an American psychologist. The principle is actually very simple; if a person behaves well, it is because he is able to do so. If a person does not behave well, it is because he cannot. At least, not in that situation. In the situation with Eric, the staff need to start examining what demands and expectations they have regarding his abilities. For each phase in the situation with Eric described above, different complex and implicit demands and expectations are involved, which must be satisfied in order for Eric to succeed in 'behaving himself'. The implicit demands and expectations in this situation are as follows:

- *Eric should be able to feel when he is hungry.* It is not uncommon for people with dementia to lose this ability.

- *Even if he can't feel that he is hungry, he should know when it's getting close to a mealtime.* Most of us know this either by keeping track of the time or by remembering when we last ate. Eric has no chance of knowing these things. He can no longer tell the time, nor can he remember when he last ate.

- *He should know that the fridge doesn't belong to him, but contains food for everyone.* Eric has lived his entire adult life in his own house with his own fridge. If the staff tell him that the fridge is not his, he can only remember it for a few minutes. His basic attitude will always be that the fridge is his and so is the food. Because that's what he's used to.

- *He should accept that it is the staff who make the decisions.* Eric has made his own decisions since he became an adult and, after all, he is in his own home (he does live in the home). The only way he will be able to understand that it is the staff who decide about the fridge is for him to simultaneously remember that it is not his fridge.

- *He should be able to delay the fulfilment of a need.* The ability to delay fulfilment of a need varies from person to person throughout life. It is what is called a *frontal function*, that is to say an ability, which requires good functioning of the frontal lobe. Eric's dementia affects, among other things, his frontal functions. This means that he is no longer able to delay need fulfilment. He is governed by impulses and can only be deterred by a new impulse, which is strong enough to block the original impulse.

- *He should understand that the staff are there for his benefit.* When Eric comes into the kitchen and is hindered by Alice, he thinks that she is trying to prevent him from taking his own food. In this situation of course he gets angry.

- *He should be able to manage anger without kicking and fighting.* This is also a so-called frontal function. Eric has always been a man with a will, and so he reacts strongly to things. Unfortunately now by hitting and kicking.

- *He should be able to regulate his affect in such a way that he does not end up in chaos and start throwing furniture around.* We can call this the ability to calm down and stay calm. We all have weak affect control in early childhood, but from the age of about 15 years, most of us are able to regulate our affect so that we don't end up in chaos. This, too, is a frontal function. Eric's dementia has unfortunately had the result that he is no longer able to control his affect as well as in the past.

- *He should be able to refuse to do what the fridge tells him to.* For Eric, the fridge has what we in dementia care call a *summoning nature*. This means that, when he sees a fridge, or when someone talks about fridges, he cannot resist opening it.

NORMAL DISTRIBUTION

Most human characteristics are distributed according to what we call 'normal distribution'. This is true of characteristics such as height, weight, intelligence, attentiveness, the ability to create structure, the ability to wait, social skills and a host of other things. Normal distribution is often illustrated as shown in Figure 2.1.

The illustration shows that most people's characteristics lie around the average. The further you move away from the average, regardless of the direction, the fewer people you will find there. This is easy to understand in relation to height, but exactly the same is true in regard to skills such as affect control, social skills, attentiveness, energy and initiative. If a person falls too far below the average in any of these characteristics, the likelihood increases that he will receive a diagnosis. But there is a gradual transition between diagnosis and normality. This means that in society there are people who handle the demands of everyday life perfectly well, many who handle them well, some who manage so-so, and a few who have great difficulty in keeping it all together.

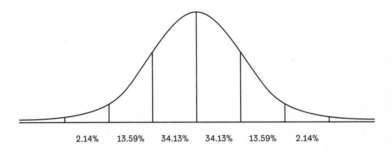

2.14%　　13.59%　　34.13%　　34.13%　　13.59%　　2.14%

Figure 2.1 The normal distribution curve

During the development of dementia, some of the affected person's characteristics will not be affected at all (such as height or vocal strength), while other characteristics will be dramatically altered. The latter are characteristics which can be said to need significant cerebral influence. We also know that the characteristics which require the most complex cognitive function are those that are most affected. This includes, for example, the ability to think while remembering, and the ability to stay attentive. Just as your memory deteriorates with age, so does your ability to handle stress and difficult situations, and this is especially true of a person with dementia. Therefore the ability to regulate affect (i.e. the ability to handle difficult situations without ending up in chaos) is lower, on average, in an 80-year-old than in a 30-year-old. This means that there are more older people than there are 30-year-olds who are unable to manage on their own in society.

And this is central to the whole philosophy on which this book is based. Every person has his own unique ability profile, and this is something that all those who work in care of older people must take into account when handling various behaviours. When we speak of behaviour that challenges, we are referring both to those who have the potential to live up to the demands we caregivers place on them, and also to those who don't. The reason that some people can't live up to demands and expectations may be deficiencies in various combinations of abilities. For example, it could be due to dementia, stress, relationships with other people in everyday life or how secure they feel, or to what extent their basic psychological needs have been fulfilled. In other words, we are not speaking about the will to behave, or about a person being well mannered or not.

Research has shown that if we use Greene's principle, 'People behave well if they can', as our point of departure, then we simply become more effective in our work. We will discuss this further in the next chapter. But first, we will consider what this principle means for daily work with behaviour that challenges.

BEHAVIOUR THAT CHALLENGES IS A PART OF EVERYDAY LIFE

Everybody working in care of older people and people with dementia will encounter situations in their daily work that get out of hand. That's just how it is. We have a tendency to consider behaviour that challenges a deviation from the norm. But really, it would be much better and more effective if we could begin to see it simply as part of everyday life. If we have the courage to study, accommodate and manage behaviour that challenges, instead of working with reprimands and demanding more medication, we will be much more effective and competent.

Each time we face a situation that has gone out of control, we should therefore sit down and think about what went wrong. In each stage of the sequence of events we will then discover exactly where we set our expectations too high. But if we then content ourselves with looking for things we think the person with the behaviour that challenges should have done differently rather than looking for the reasons that actually lay behind the behaviour, we will face the same problem next time we end up in a similar situation.

DEMANDS AND EXPECTATIONS

So what we need to do then, is to sit down and consider our own behaviour and our own expectations of a certain person's abilities, and compare them with the person's real abilities, especially when dealing with someone with dementia. Then it won't be so hard to understand. If a person behaves in a negative way, we are sure to find something that we have done wrong. Admittedly it demands a great deal of us as professionals to see ourselves and our own role in relation to the people with dementia that we work with. At the same time it is essential, if we are to avoid the same situation arising again and again. Because all the behaviour they exhibit occurs in interplay with their surroundings. Either in direct interaction with those of us who work in homes for older people, or in an interaction with the physical framework over which we have control.

In order to have a long-term and solid basis for evaluation and planning in regard to behaviour that challenges, we should reflect on the demands and expectations we are placing on older individuals' abilities:

- *The ability to calculate cause and effect in complex situations.* This is needed in order to foresee the consequences of one's own actions, but also in order to form an idea of what is likely to happen in a more general sense. People who have difficulty with this need much more structure and predictability than others do. Some people (nearly 20% of the population) have problems with this function throughout their lives. This is a complex ability that people quickly lose upon the development of dementia.

- *The ability to start, structure, plan and perform activities.* These are classic frontal functions, which are often considerably affected upon the development of dementia. Furthermore, this ability is dependent on the working memory, that you know what you are doing, how far you have come, and when you are finished. This means that we can't expect people with dementia to be able to organise, plan and carry out activities. Instead, they need support in the form of a structure that they can see and relate to, or that we can support them with along the way.

- *The ability to carry out a concrete action.* Many people with dementia develop *apraxia*. This means that practical skills and the ability to carry out actions automatically disappear. All of a sudden, you can no longer dress yourself, because you can't button your shirt, or can't remember in what order things should be done. Does the underwear go on first or last?

- *The ability to process sensory impressions and to understand the world.* It is easy to assume that people with dementia perceive the world in the same way as everyone else.

But the truth is that their brain injuries often make it difficult for them to understand, recognise and interpret what they see and hear, which leads to misinterpretations in everyday life. A toothbrush may be mistaken for a hairbrush, for example. Generally the senses also deteriorate, which further reduces this ability.

- *The ability to understand what other people are saying.* This ability is often weakened upon the development of dementia. Sometimes it is obvious that no language skills remain, and then we have to resort to non-verbal communication. At other times, we may be fooled into having too high expectations, for example when a person is socially competent and succeeds in getting through conversations with the help of platitudes. He may perhaps use the same ten phrases the whole time ('yes, that's true', 'that's good then', 'you don't say?') But the person may still not really understand what we are talking about.

- *The ability to express oneself verbally.* Most of us have a tendency to listen to what people say, and not how they say it. If a person with dementia has difficulty in expressing himself, perhaps we don't bother speaking with him. We may think that the person isn't very sociable, only saying 'yes' or 'no', but on closer inspection discover that he is actually unable to express himself.

- *The ability to remember while thinking.* This ability is also called *working memory*. Many people with dementia are unable to remember something and at the same time process the information they have in their head. In this case, spoken instructions are useless. Instead, we have to provide support throughout an entire activity, through personal assistance, lists or the like. We can also provide support by stimulating several senses simultaneously, for example by telling the person he is going to shower (hearing) while at the same time holding out a towel (sight). Or by creating a strong smell of food by frying a little bacon just before lunch is served. Even if bacon is not on the menu that day.

- *The ability to think quickly.* Most people with dementia have slow processing speed and so can only concentrate on one thing at a time and at their own pace. If we are going to show the person what to do, we must do so slowly enough to be sure that he can keep up.

- *The ability to divide your attention.* For example, it may be difficult for a person with dementia to hear what we are trying to say if the TV is on at the same time, because he can only focus his attention on one thing at a time.

- *The ability to remember and learn.* Even though we are working with people with diminished memory skills, strangely enough we often still expect them to remember exactly what we have said or to learn to do things they couldn't do before. The great majority of people with dementia cannot remember what happened yesterday, or what is going to happen on the weekend or next week. They can get around this problem to some extent, however, if we let their body learn subconsciously instead, for example by repeatedly walking the same route with them over to the day centre. That they can remember this with their body does not mean that they can show someone else the way to the day centre. It's not a conscious knowledge. But in this way we can use physical knowledge to get their everyday life work for them. We can even initiate an action (that is physically remembered) such as going to the toilet by showing them the toilet.

- *The ability to resist impulses.* Many people with dementia react directly to what is happening in the immediate situation and are simply unable to refrain from reacting once an impulse is felt. We must therefore consider what impulses we have created through rules and the way we treat people. Rules about what a person must not do often create the impulse to do just that.

- *Endurance.* Some people find it much more difficult than others to wait. They also have difficulty in doing things that require prolonged concentration. This is partly because the ability to focus is strongly affected, and partly because the ability to delay need-fulfilment is diminished. With the development of dementia, the ability to wait is often very strongly affected. So waiting can be very difficult.

- *The ability to be flexible or to re-adjust quickly.* Most people actually prefer when things remain the same way as usual. However, some people with dementia find it extremely difficult to adjust to any change, even if the change is necessary, and even if we think they should be able to cope with it. People with diminished flexibility end up in conflict with others more often than people who are more flexible.

- *The ability to gauge other people's thoughts, feelings and actions, so-called social competence.* Some people with dementia lose the ability to see their own role in situations that go wrong or to understand how situations and actions are experienced by others. They therefore often find it very difficult to gauge other people's intentions. They don't know what we want. Social competence is strongly affected in frontotemporal dementia. We see problems with social competence in other dementia illnesses also, but in these cases it may be the case that the affected person always lacked social skills. Unfortunately, when a person with dementia moves in with a number of other people in a care home, the demands and expectations of social competence are greatly increased. This is something that very well may lead to behaviour that challenges. For many people, however, their social skills are not affected at all, and this may be the only ability that they retain well into the course of their dementia. This means that they can participate in social events and receive great pleasure from them, but it can also sometimes lead to underestimation of their difficulties.

- *The ability to feel empathy or to see another person's perspective.* This is an ability which is often diminished in people with dementia. This can be a direct effect of the brain injury caused by the dementia. But it can also be a result of the difficulty these people have in coping with others when they are having a really tough time themselves. To see a situation from someone else's perspective is an extremely complex function and is often impossible for a damaged brain. In spite of this, we often find ourselves expecting these people to understand that we also have to care for the other residents in our department, or that we are busy and that means they have to wait for a while. Maybe this idea of showing consideration for others is so ingrained in us that it seems provocative or antisocial when someone doesn't do it. But it's not out of selfishness or meanness that people with dementia fail to understand other people's perspective. It is their brain injury that makes them unable to behave correctly.

- *The ability to handle stress.* People can take varying amounts of stress. But, generally speaking, we become more sensitive to stress as we grow older, and the development of dementia most often increases this tendency.

- *The ability to say 'yes'.* It sounds strange, but some people say 'yes' to most things in life, and some say 'no'. This is a personal characteristic that is not easily changed. If a person with dementia has difficulty in saying 'yes', then we need to increase his level of participation by, for example, giving him options to choose from or by asking in different ways so that we can get a feel for what the person wants. Also, the development of dementia increases the risk that a person will say 'no', because we humans often say 'no' to things we don't understand. We must therefore investigate the 'noes' we receive by trying again in different ways. The person may be saying 'no' because he really doesn't want to (and is thereby exercising his right to self-determination), but it may also be because he doesn't fully understand the question. It may also be good to ask a slow processor the same question several times. Then he will have time to think.

- *The ability to regulate affect.* This ability is about how we humans calm down or stay calm. This ability varies from person to person and improves with age, up to adulthood.

But it deteriorates again when you start to grow old. Particularly in people with frontal injury, it gets continuously worse. It's important to understand that this is an ability, it's not a matter of will. No-one wants to lose control over their feelings.

It is important for us to be aware of all the abilities listed above. In addition, we must lower the demands and expectations we have that people with dementia should have the same level of ability every day or every hour. What they are able to do and what we can expect from them will vary, depending among other things on the time of day and the level of stress. It is difficult to know whether Greene's mantra 'People behave well if they can' is true. But it's effective. That's enough for us. If all of us who work in older and dementia care think this way, the amount of conflict will fall – a lot. It will also have the result that the people with dementia who we work with will be happy and develop, and that our own feeling of success will increase. But to get there, we need to adapt our work according to the abilities that each individual possesses. This doesn't mean that we necessarily need more staff, but rather that we plan our work with the individual as point of departure.

Summary
When a person with dementia exhibits behaviour that challenges it is most often because we have too high expectations of their abilities. In order to reduce behaviour that challenges we must therefore identify where it is that our expectations are too high. Because people with dementia always do the very best they can.

3

People Always Do What Makes Sense

ANNA

Anna has lived in the care home for five years. During the past year she has had increasing difficulties with her memory. It is common for the staff to find her in another resident's room. As a rule, Anna is quite happy to leave with the staff when asked to do so.

On this particular afternoon, nursing aide Susan is asked to come to Bill's room. At the door, Susan meets Bill's daughter, who is very upset and says: 'It's scandalous that you can't keep better watch over your residents. There's a strange woman lying in my father's bed and if you don't get her out at once, or if it happens again, I will file a complaint!'

Susan goes over to the bed and takes hold of Anna while explaining: 'Anna, this is not your bed and you can't lie here, come at once or Bill will be very angry.' Anna pulls her arm away and says: 'Leave me alone, you stupid girl, I'm tired and this is my husband. Go away!' Susan fetches a colleague and together they remove Anna forcefully from Bill's room.

ACTIONS THAT MAKE SENSE

We humans do what is most meaningful to us in any given situation. Regardless of whether we have a dementia illness or not. We create meaning by weighing impressions and memories. So does Anna. Anna can no longer understand spatial relationships – a common difficulty in Alzheimer-type dementia. So she often goes wrong. When she enters a room such as Bill's, she navigates the best she can. She creates meaning and makes the situation understandable for herself. Because that's what we humans do. The meaning she creates is presumably that she is at home with her husband. That's not such a dumb meaning. She did live together with her husband for many years, and so the situation is familiar to her. Susan and the other staff members don't know how Bill is taking it. But they do know that his daughter is upset. Because Anna's behaviour doesn't make sense to her. And the staff are also having a hard time making the situation make sense. So Susan first asks Anna to leave the room, and when Anna doesn't want to do so, she gets help from a colleague and forces her out.

This doesn't make any sense to Anna. She's in a familiar and meaningful situation, convinced that she is resting at home together with her husband of the same age. When Susan asks her to leave the room, Anna thinks she wants to throw her out of her own home. Of course she doesn't want to agree to this. Anna resists. Because it makes sense.

We all do what makes sense to us in any given situation. For example, we drive more slowly if there is a speed bump in the road or if the road twists and turns than if the road is good, wide and smooth. Usually without really thinking about it. In other words our behaviour in traffic is guided by the road.

To retreat from a situation that demands too much of our abilities is fully understandable. It is actually the most sensible thing to do. Similarly, it makes sense that Anna is comfortable in the familiar and therefore meaningful situation of resting together with a man of the same age.

Meaningfulness and sense are not about understanding. It's common for staff to think that they can change people's behaviour simply by talking with them. We don't think so. 'You must surely understand...' is not the way to proceed when a person does not have the ability to calculate cause and effect in complex situations. Neither is it meaningful for a staff member to explain why he doesn't have time to help a person just now, if that person is no longer very good at seeing things from someone else's perspective.

WHAT RULES SHOULD WE HAVE?

One of the most common examples of behaviour that challenges is when someone doesn't follow the rules. This can be very provoking, because it is deeply ingrained in us that rules must be obeyed. Neither is it unusual, when a problem arises, that the first thing we do is to introduce a new rule. But if we take a closer look at ourselves we will discover that we don't obey all the rules in society either. We obey the rules that make sense. We have trouble obeying rules that don't.

This is easy to see in traffic. For example, we are more likely to drive within the speed limit in an old car than if we have a new car in which the sensation of speed is less evident. And we may walk through a red light if there is no traffic. In the same way, people with dementia follow the rules that make sense and cheat with the ones that don't.

Rules about smoking are problematic. In many care homes, smoking is not allowed in communal spaces. But to someone who has smoked all his life and who believes that he is in his own home, this rule may not make sense. If the staff then demand that the person obeys this rule, it can lead to daily conflict. This kind of situation can ruin what we call the alliance, which is the cornerstone of all care provision. Not for all the residents, but for those who are smokers.

It is therefore extremely important to carefully consider which rules should apply at the home where we work. Because rules that don't make sense to older people only undermine the quality of our work. Rules that we stick to simply to show our authority or power have a directly negative effect on both the alliance and on older residents' quality of life. What is needed, then, is to retain the rules that older people are familiar with from their own lives and which they will obey without question. But also to do away with the rules that we find don't work.

Rules are also something people with dementia must learn to remember if they are to work. But people with dementia are not very good at learning things, nor do they remember very well. So generally speaking, rules are very difficult in dementia care.

THE PHYSICAL ENVIRONMENT IS IMPORTANT

If we want to work with sense and meaning as a pedagogical principle, there are a number of shortcuts available. It's always good to start by looking at the physical environment, for example. 'Building away' behaviour that challenges is often the cheapest solution. By this we mean that it is important to have a well-functioning physical framework and to understand how the residents' sensory needs are affected by their physical environment. It is therefore important to think about the following:

- *We are affected by colour, light, space and sound.* Soft light without hard contrasts makes us calm. For this reason it's a good idea to have light coming from two directions in communal rooms and other spaces where stress levels are elevated. It is also important to make sure that there is plenty of space available in situations that require it. Many conflicts arise, for example, when we accompany someone to the bathroom or help someone put their outdoor clothes on in the entrance hall, where conditions are cramped. Adding a little space reduces both the level of noise and the level of conflict. A door that doesn't make a loud noise when slammed shut but quietly glides into place also creates calm. Furthermore, soft, somewhat subdued colours are generally more helpful in lowering stress levels than strong ones. Unnecessary noise should also obviously be avoided. It is usually quiet and peaceful in most care homes. Older people don't always hear very well. Yet it's still a good idea to soundproof properly. Almost but not quite hearing what someone is saying is more likely to create anxiety and paranoia than not hearing at all that someone is speaking. Especially if you don't really know what's going on, or where you are.

- *We are governed by the physical environment.* Most of us would rather walk down a wide passage than a narrow one, for example, and rather open a light-coloured door than a dark one. And if there's an echo, some people whistle more. This means that a care home should have good, muted acoustics (if we want a peaceful environment) with dark doors to the rooms where we don't want the older people to go and wide, light-coloured doors to the rooms where we do want them to go. If there is a wide door leading outside that they shouldn't go through then it needs to be disguised a little, perhaps by making it part of a mural. Many people with dementia have difficulty interpreting visual input. This means that they may think a black doormat is a hole. A black doormat in front of a door that we don't want them to go through can therefore be an excellent idea.

- *The requirements on the physical environment increase when it is people with dementia who live there.* That they can easily find their way around is important. The ability to understand spatial relationships is strongly affected in people with Alzheimer-type dementia and commonly affected in other types of dementia. These people have difficulty in understanding where they are, and can't find the way to where they are going. By building in such a way that they can see where to go, we make things easier for them. Therefore, labyrinth-like and preferably also multi-storey buildings should be avoided. Rather, it is important that lines of sight are clear and kept free of clutter, while still striving to provide a setting that is as homelike and pleasant as possible. Overly-large rooms should also be avoided, because they can feel overwhelming. It is also a good idea to avoid glass walls and glass doors. Glass that goes all the way to the floor is often interpreted as a doorway by people with dementia. Windows at normal height are to be preferred, even if in a door.

- *People are positively affected by a familiar environment.* Care homes are workplaces and therefore often furnished in such a way that they can easily be kept clean. They seldom resemble a home, usually being more institutional in nature. Because of this, people with dementia may have a hard time feeling at home. They may think they are in a hospital or a communal building. In the 1990s, a care home in Sweden was furnished with furniture from the 1940s and this was observed to have a good effect on the well-being of the residents. Unfortunately, for reasons of hygiene and the work environment, it was necessary to revert to using more practical furniture. In the UK, creative staff at a care home have tried to solve the problem by creating kernels of recognition for the residents. They have some cars from the 1940s and 1950s, for example, which were common when the residents were young adults. If someone is restless a member of staff will take them for a drive. This usually helps. In order to keep up with the times, they now also have some cars from the 1960s and 1970s. Similarly, the residential home for people with dementia, Pilehuset, in Copenhagen has a shopping street in the cellar. The floor of the corridor has been painted black, with white lines down the middle and sidewalks, and the rooms have display windows. Here they can buy soft drinks, cookies and cakes in Mrs Hansen's cellar, or articles of hygiene in Schou's Perfumery, they can drink a beer at 'The Rat Hole', visit the toy museum or pick up activity materials at the exchange centre. The staff have to fetch all activity materials in the shopping street and can only go there in the company of a resident. In this way, isles of familiarity are created for older people.

CREATE SENSE THROUGH PREDICTABILITY

Another shortcut we can use when working with making sense and meaning as the pedagogical principle is to create sense through predictability. For example, many people with dementia have no trouble remaining quiet and calm if they have an overview of what they are going to do and for how long. For people who no longer understand the concept of time, for example, it may work to have activities with a clear finish. It is easier for them to understand that they should wash dishes until they are done than to understand that they should wait for ten minutes. Washing dishes is a familiar, predictable and understandable activity with a clear end.

A familiar activity is predictable in itself. For example, Tom Kitwood has described how people with dementia, when presented with a basket full of hand towels, will often fold the towels. Folding towels is something most of them have done all their lives. Nearly everyone knows how to do it. This makes the activity something they can do for an extended period of time. It also makes the activity meaningful for them. Not in the sense that it's meaningful to fold the towels. That's only important for us who know that they need to be folded. But when one's world is becoming fragmentary and unpredictable, it's good to do something that is practical and familiar.

Most older people have lived a long life where the daily routine was similar on most days of the week. Continuing with this routine is another example of a good way to create predictability. In the situation with Anna described at the beginning of the chapter, this could mean that she eats her dinner at five-thirty just as she has done for most of her life. Whereas her fellow-resident, Charles, perhaps prefers to eat at six, because that's what he's used to. If Anna has to wait until six she gets anxious and starts looking for the staff. If Charles gets his dinner at five-thirty, he may not be able to make sense of his day. Five-thirty for him could just as well be two-thirty. But six o'clock is familiar and predictable.

Many people with dementia lose their sense of time, but this doesn't mean they lose awareness of what they used to do in the afternoon. This means that we may very well be able to use vague indications of time to create meaning for them. For example, we can say: 'Would you like to take a little nap now after lunch?' And when they show up again after half an hour: 'We'll have our afternoon coffee in about an hour.' Even if the person won't know when an hour has passed and most likely will have forgotten all about it, it's still reassuring to hear that it's soon time for afternoon coffee, when you've just woken up and perhaps don't quite know whether it's morning or evening.

Summary
People don't always act rationally. We do what makes sense in the situation in which we find ourselves. This means that we are influenced by a host of different factors every time we do something. By influencing these factors we can change a person's behaviour. In dementia, we have to take a little extra care about which factors we change.

4

Those Who Take Responsibility Can Make a Difference

MYRTLE

At a staff meeting, the group working evenings every other week says that Myrtle is causing a lot of trouble. They usually find her very wound up. She runs around after them and follows them into all the different rooms, to the point where it's just impossible for them to do their job. They argue that the day staff should make sure she calms down before the evening shift starts, and suggest that they take her for a walk to tire her out or, alternatively, give her some calming medication. A long discussion ensues, where the day staff don't consider it their problem since they don't find Myrtle wound up, and besides, they don't have time to take her for walks. The second group of evening staff that alternates weeks with the first group reports that Myrtle likes to help them wash the dishes after supper and evening coffee. When she has finished the dishes, she sits down, drinks a cup of coffee, and nods off. The first group of evening staff really don't see this is a potential solution for their weeks; they work in a different way and can't give special consideration to Myrtle.

WHO IS RESPONSIBLE?

The principle 'Those who take responsibility can make a difference' was formulated by psychologist Bernhard Weiner in 1995. It was very widely spread within the field of occupational psychology, where concepts such as *influencing one's own work environment* became important in order to reduce sick-leave and increase job satisfaction. In care circles, it is the psychologist Dave Dagnan who has carried Weiner's idea the furthest. He has looked a little into how staff caring for older people perceive their behaviour, and how the staff's views on the extent to which the older people control their own behaviour influence the effectiveness of the care they provide. In the example described above, a member of the evening shifts feels that Myrtle should be calm. If she isn't, it's either the day staff's fault (they didn't tire her out) or Myrtle's own fault (she isn't tired enough and so needs calming medication).

When we handle a situation in this way, placing the responsibility on the older person or on other staff, we are making ourselves powerless. Then we have no possibility of resolving the situation. And powerless personnel without the ability to make a difference is a big problem and the wrong way to go if we want to reduce behaviour that challenges.

In his research, Dave Dagnan has studied what happens when, for example, members of staff think that older people are intentionally causing trouble, as compared to thinking that they are doing their best but not succeeding. The results are amazing. If we stick to the example of Myrtle, then first of all, if the evening staff held Myrtle responsible for her own behaviour, they would experience many similar situations. Second, they would have a feeling of impotence about being able to influence Myrtle's behaviour. This means that they would go to work each day in fear and trepidation of how badly things may go. It could get to the point that it depended on Myrtle whether the evening staff have a good shift or not. Circumstances such as these lead to increased absence due to illness and a greater turnover of staff. This in turn has a negative effect on the well-being of the residents.

If, on the other hand, the evening staff decided that Myrtle was doing her best, but that the situation was too unstructured for her to navigate in, then they could have created a familiar and understandable situation for her. They would then have been able to avoid the same problem occurring again and at the same time would have received the ability to influence the situation and, by extension, their work environment. This would mean fewer days off sick, reduced staff turnover, and better quality of life for Myrtle and the other residents.

Instead of giving Myrtle sedative medication, the staff should find out what they themselves can do to reduce her behaviour that challenges. For example, by considering how the other evening shift solves the problem by allowing her to wash dishes, something she finds meaningful, familiar and understandable. But they should also take a look at their own role: why is sedative medication the first thing they think of when they run into a problem at work? As members of staff, how can they become proficient at first seeing what they themselves can do? Here we can use the same thought process that we did with Eric, who hit and kicked staff member Alice in order to get to the fridge. It's easy to say what he should have done, but harder to get him to do it. He does what is most meaningful to him in the situation, which is to hit and kick. If Alice wants to change the situation, then she needs to find out what she can do to bring about such a change.

PUNISHMENT AND CONSEQUENCES

This way of thinking may seem provocative since it is contrary to the usual ideas about power relationships and relationships between people with dementia and staff. One objection might be: 'Should he really be allowed to act like that? Shouldn't there be consequences?' This objection is interesting for several reasons. In the first place, probably no-one thinks it's OK for Eric to hit people or throw furniture around. Not even Eric. But in a difficult situation, he does the best he can. Things go the way they do. And that's what the staff have to relate to. So the question then is what can be done to reduce the risk of it happening again. This is where consequences come in. Most people think that if you suffer a negative consequence after behaving in a certain way, then you are less likely to behave that way again. Because that's how we think it works with us. In psychological thinking, we see this as learning. If it works, that is. But this way of thinking meets with certain difficulties when it comes to dementia. Dementia involves a loss of skills, among others the ability to learn. So, even if such a method for handling negative behaviour worked for normal people, it wouldn't work for people with dementia.

In addition to this, the difference between punishment and functioning consequences has been debated by psychologists, sociologists and educators for many a year. If we look at all the available research, there is really only one factor of interest: if a person perceives a negative consequence as a punishment, the problem behaviour is more likely to increase than to decrease. In other words, the important thing is not what actually happens but how it is perceived by the person. The consequences that we remember and that we feel were of help to us are not those that we perceived as punishment. For a consequence to work, the person affected must be able both to learn from it and to see it in a context that gives it meaning. It must not be perceived as a punishment. Unfortunately, however, the chances of people with dementia managing this are extremely small. Therefore they will most often perceive consequences as unpredictable punishment. And about this we know a great deal:

- We know, for example, that punishment usually results in a person feeling unfairly treated. And feeling unfairly treated by the staff means a thorn in the relationship.

- We also know that punishment increases the very behaviour that is being punished. This is true both on the societal and the individual level. This is the reason why first-offence criminals often receive conditional sentences. An unconditional sentence for a first offence results in a 150 per cent higher recurrence rate compared with a conditional sentence.

- We know, too, that punishment can legitimise behaviour that challenges. Research by Gneezy and Rutichini has shown that you can double the number of children still at a day care centre at closing time if you institute fines for parents who pick up their children late. The reason is that the punishment removes the bad conscience. If you're willing to pay what it costs, you don't need to have a bad conscience. This effect works both ways. If you know what it will cost, there's a risk that you consider the value of the action higher than the price you have to pay. Then you will perform the action. It may also be the case that if you are punished for your action, then you no longer feel you have to think about the fact that what you did was wrong. After all, you took your punishment!

- Another effect of punishment can be called the de Quervain effect, after the Swiss neurophysiologist Dominique de Quervain, who published an interesting article in 2005. Together with some colleagues he investigated two things: partly whether there are differences between people who punish, and partly why we punish others. They arrived at some interesting answers. First, that people's tendency to punish others differs. Second, that it is possible to predict this tendency by measuring activity in an area of the brain called the dorsal striatum. The greater the activity in this area when a person is punishing someone, the greater that person's tendency to punish will be. In other words, there are biological differences between people who like to punish and those who are reluctant to do so. So for the staff, it is important to take their own proclivities into account here, since punishment doesn't have any positive effect on the punished person's behaviour. But the most interesting aspect of Dominique de Quervain's study is why we punish others. The researchers showed that a person who is punishing another receives a personal feeling of being competent. So even if the person loses something by punishing another, he still gets a feeling of competence and justice.

  There has been speculation into why this is so. One of those with a theory is the American anthropologist Robert Boyd. He thinks that in prehistoric times, people who got rid of those who were spoiling things for the flock or village by throwing them out before they could do too much damage survived better than those who did not. This is the reason, according to him, why we have developed a reward effect when we punish others. In a care home, however, the objective is to get the residents to have a good life, even though they are no longer very good at looking after themselves. Here the survival of the staff is not at stake if a person doesn't behave well.

The question then is not whether a person with dementia, such as Eric or Myrtle, should be permitted to say or do the things they do. The question is rather how we can make sure they don't do it again. And then we are back at the principle in the earlier chapter, 'People behave well if they can'. What was it in Myrtle's situation that she couldn't cope with? In a similar situation, how could we change the circumstances so that things would go better next time?

THE SKILL CEILING

As staff, we are good at taking responsibility when we have a good method. When we know what to do and what works, we do it willingly. But sometimes we find ourselves in situations where we lack a method that works. We lack appropriate skills. We can call this *hitting the skill ceiling*. In such situations, we have a tendency to immediately pass the responsibility on to someone else.

Perhaps we place the responsibility on the older person by punishing him (with the argument that 'maybe then he'll learn; after all, he has to take responsibility'), by asking for sedative medication, or by shouting, yelling and scolding. Perhaps we sometimes think, 'he has to behave, and if he doesn't understand that, I'll say it again, but louder so that he understands'.

Another example could be that we shift the responsibility to our manager or to the politicians. This we can do by saying: 'This man's behaviour is so bad that he shouldn't be in a regular care home. He should be in a hospital.' And certainly, there may be some people who need more support than others. Only it doesn't help them to be admitted to a psychiatric ward. So when we think that a person shouldn't be allowed to stay in a normal care home, it seldom has to do with his needs, but more often with our own unwillingness or inability to make the adjustments necessary for him to manage in his normal environment. By learning to adjust ourselves and our work to an individual person's needs, we take responsibility, and thereby gain the opportunity to make a difference.

There is also a tendency for us to explain a resident's behaviour by the behaviour of his relatives, and to put the responsibility on them. But if we want to succeed in our assignment we have to adjust our methods rather than talking about difficult relatives. That doesn't help us in our mission, it only makes us stop trying. And then we are really betraying those in our care. Difficult relatives increase both our responsibility and our work load. They do not reduce the requirement to succeed.

Finally, we may have a tendency to lay the responsibility for behaviour that we find difficult to manage on our co-workers. In the example about Myrtle, one of the evening crew blames the day crew for not doing their job. They think the day crew should go for walks with Myrtle. Every time we suggest what someone else can do to solve our problem in this way, we are relinquishing our responsibility. But also our possibility to make a difference. Sometimes it gets absurd. Such as when one group of staff thinks they have a problem because another group works in a different way. But what if the other group doesn't have a problem? Why should they then adjust and work in the same way as the group that does have a problem? If we have a problem, we must always find out what we ourselves can do to change the situation.

If we are to succeed then, we must realise when we have reached our skill ceiling. This is perhaps one of the most important tasks we have as members of staff. We can use a simple rule of thumb. If we are using the same methods our parents used with us when we were kids, we are probably going the wrong way about it. The reason is simple. We are professionals. Our parents were not, in their relationship with us. They were actually amateurs. Just like we ourselves are when raising our kids. Our parents could bring up fairly normal children. But we couldn't expect them to take on people with dementia. This means that if we are using their methods we shouldn't be getting paid. Because then we're acting as amateurs.

A simple way of testing whether we have reached the skill ceiling is to use a principle often but incorrectly attributed to Albert Einstein: 'Insanity is doing the same thing over and over again and expecting a different result.' One way to recognise when we have reached the skill ceiling, then, is to count. Have we tried this several times before? Did it work then? If it didn't work before, why are we doing it again? Is there any chance that it will work better this time?

Because if we reach the skill ceiling and start placing the responsibility for the behaviour of residents such as Myrtle or Eric on them, on our bosses and politicians, or on relatives or colleagues, then we will lose the possibility to influence their behaviour. This will make us ineffective, sick days will probably increase, and the risk that we suffer a breakdown will increase greatly.

Summary

If we want to change something, we have to think of what we ourselves can do to bring about the change. Not what others should do. Only by investigating what we can do ourselves can we influence the course of events. This implies that we who work in care of older people should focus on what we ourselves can do and accept our responsibility. Not lay the responsibility on the residents, their relatives, colleagues or managers.

5

People With Dementia No Longer Learn

CHARLIE

Charlie is sitting with the newspaper at the table in the lounge after lunch. It is quiet, since many of the other residents have gone off to their rooms. This is the best part of the day for Charlie. Then two staff members, Hannah and Jane, arrive and sit down at the table. Jane has a bag of toffees and she offers one to Charlie. The wrapper lands on the floor. Hannah, who is sitting opposite Charlie, points her finger at him and tells him to pick up the wrapper. Charlie looks up for a moment and then back down at the newspaper. Jane then points at the wrapper on the floor and asks Charlie: 'What's that on the floor?' Hannah holds up the bag in front of Charlie and says: 'You can have another one if you pick it up.' Charlie looks at her for a long time, then gets up and goes off to his room. When the night staff come in, they ask where Charlie is, since he is usually sitting at the table and greets them when they arrive.

MEMORY, LEARNING AND CONSEQUENCES

The principle 'People with dementia no longer learn' should not be surprising. Dementia is usually described as a memory disorder, and it is quite logical that memory and learning go together. But things still often go wrong. Situations like the one described above unfortunately occur all the time in care of older people. Since Charlie is the one who dropped the wrapper, Hannah and Jane think that he should be the one to pick it up. Similar situations arise when something has been spilt. The one who spilled should be the one to clean it up.

If we had asked Hannah and Jane why they acted like they did, there are some different answers that we might have received:

- Charlie should pick up the wrapper because he's the one who dropped it. We must all take responsibility for our actions.

- Charlie should pick up the wrapper so that he learns not to throw paper around everywhere.

- Charlie should pick up the wrapper in order to maintain his level of functioning.

The first answer is absurd. Charlie lives in a care home because he is unable to take responsibility for himself. Besides, he's an old man with a body that is not as flexible as it used to be. The effort it would take for him to pick up the wrapper is many times greater than the effort it would take for Hannah or Jane to do it. Furthermore, they are paid to be there, he is not.

In our discussions with staff working in older care, some have been extremely provoked when we answered them in the way described above. They then often end up at the next answer instead. But this is even more absurd. A person like Charlie lives in a care home because he has dementia. He no longer learns things. Even if he does pick up the wrapper it doesn't mean he won't throw it on the floor the next time he is given a toffee.

Hannah and Jane's third conceivable answer builds on the idea of everyday occupational therapy that is currently very common in the dementia field. The basic idea is that the staff's foremost task is to give help to self-help. By getting Charlie to be active, Hannah and Jane would be helping him to support and thereby maintain his level of functioning. The idea of activating Charlie is good, but it is then also necessary to get him to think that picking up the wrapper is meaningful. Simply telling him what to do is not providing help to self-help. And there is definitely no self-determination involved.

WE CANNOT TEACH PEOPLE WITH DEMENTIA HOW TO BEHAVE

When Charlie grew up, his parents no longer made decisions for him. Since then, he has made his own decisions. He has taken responsibility for his own life and decided by himself when he wants decisions made for him. All the power relationships he has entered into, as an employee and as a citizen, have been regulated by law. Because that's how it works. When he eventually moved into a care home, it wasn't because he became a child again. It was because he needed help to cope with his everyday life. For the rest of his life, Charlie will presumably need more and more help with each passing day. Maybe even to remove the wrapper from the toffee and to put it in his mouth. But for now he can manage that part himself. What he can't do now is to handle both the paper and the toffee properly. And he can't understand why he should have to pick up a piece of paper that's lying on the floor.

It is not the staff's job to go back to an earlier stage in Charlie's development and start bringing him up again. Upbringing is something they can do in their own time with their own children. Children. There is an important difference here. They can make decisions for their children because they are still children. Children have to learn how to take responsibility for themselves. When they become sensible adults, they can make decisions for themselves. But Charlie isn't going to learn anything at all. Nor is he going to take responsibility for himself. He has been able to do this for most of his life. So the fact that he can't do so any more is not because he hasn't yet learnt how.

WHAT DOES A REPRIMAND REALLY DO?

There is another important factor at play in the situation with the toffee wrapper. That the staff are handing out a reprimand. Neuropsychologist Anna van Duijvenvoorde and her colleagues in Leiden in the Netherlands conducted an interesting research project in 2008. Not actually on people with dementia, but the project is still of interest to mention. The researchers measured brain activity in children and adults during various activities, using an MRI camera. In the experiment, each participant was given a number of tasks to solve. But they were not told how to solve them. If they solved a problem well, they received praise of the type 'That was right.' When they were wrong, they were told 'That was wrong.' The researchers were interested in finding out whether the test subjects learned from success or from failure.

The results were totally unexpected. When a normal, well-functioning adult was told: 'That was wrong', the level of activity increased in the parts of the brain that have to do with learning. On the other hand, if the same person was told, 'That was right', the level of activity in the same areas diminished considerably. When the same experiment was done with children, the opposite result was seen. When the children were told that they were right, the brain activity increased, and when they heard that they were wrong, it decreased.

This then implies that well-functioning adults learn from failures, while children learn from success. In the 13–15 years age group, the results varied a bit from child to child, which the researchers took to mean that this is the age at which a child develops from learning through success to learning through failure. The theory is that we humans learn from deviations from the norm. Normal children fail the whole time when they are young. As they grow older they get better and better and, sometime before they turn 15, most of them succeed more often than they fail.

When little, children are surprised when they succeed; as adults, we are surprised when we fail. This is one of the reasons why many people give up a sport or stop playing a musical instrument around the age of 13–15. Suddenly we discover that we are not particularly good. Only those who are really good at something keep on with it. This also means that, as adults, we are not particularly surprised when someone tells us that we are good at something. Although we may be somewhat embarrassed and unsure of how to reply. Correspondingly, children are not surprised when something they do goes wrong. Because it doesn't come as a surprise to them.

Admittedly this research is not about older people. But the theory can easily be extrapolated to people with dementia.

Because what happens during the progress of dementia is that a person fails more and more often in what they are trying to do. This makes them gradually lose their self-confidence and they start to expect to fail. This early stage of the development of dementia in particular is often full of anxiety. The person's world is collapsing around them and they are worried about how it will all end. Eventually the anxiety disappears for most people because they no longer have the ability to compare with what they once were able to do. But they no longer expect to succeed, and so they are not surprised when they fail.

The fact that a person is used to failure doesn't mean that his self-confidence is unaffected when it happens, however. Even late in the course of their illness, a person with dementia is still affected by failure and can say things like, 'Do I have to be here' and 'I can't, help me.' To then reprimand that person is to put focus on their failure. And that has a negative effect on both their well-being and self-confidence.

But the most important thing about van Duijvenvoorde's research is that she is speaking about learning. She is able to show that both the stick and the carrot have to do with learning. We praise or reprimand people in order for them to learn. But people with dementia are no longer able to learn. After all, learning builds on remembering something. This doesn't mean that we shouldn't give praise and compliments to people with dementia. Because praise and compliments create a good atmosphere and that is central to all work with people, especially people who live in the present and whose well-being and quality of life depend on the prevailing mood.

There is thus no reason to reprimand people with dementia. It simply has no effect. On the contrary, reprimands lead only to bad temper and directly affect the person's well-being and the quality of life that it is our primary task to secure.

SETTING LIMITS

It is fashionable today to speak of setting limits. Politicians do it in regard to criminals or when discussing various expressions of culture, and most of us do it when we speak of raising children.

Setting boundaries is a special way of saying 'Stop' in order to prevent or interrupt a behaviour. A behaviour can be prevented or interrupted in many ways. Some are positive and work well in the situation (we will look at these shortly). However the method of 'setting limits' absolutely does not work. It involves mixing learning into the situation we are trying to prevent.

BENNY

Benny is perceived by the staff as boundary-crossing and perverse. He is very interested in the women in the home and likes to sit close to them. He strokes their hair and tries to kiss them and sometimes follows them into their rooms. One day when he is sitting in the lounge, the staff see him with his hand in his pants, which they take to mean that he is rubbing his penis while watching the women. One of the staff, Christina, quickly goes over to him and says: 'Benny, stop that, we don't do that kind of thing here.'

Benny looks at her in confusion and carries on. Christina then yanks Benny's hand away to get him to understand. Benny still looks confused but doesn't restart the behaviour.

In this situation, setting a limit involves Christina telling Benny to stop what he is doing. But she also includes an expectation of learning in what she says. Because she says: 'We don't do that kind of thing here.' This is a completely meaningless thing to say in a conversation with a person with dementia; it is based on the idea that Benny can remember what Christina has said the next time he has the same impulse.

It is reasonable to assume that Benny has managed in social situations throughout his adult life without putting his hand in his pants. But now he no longer can. He is no longer very good at preventing himself. By this we don't mean to say that all men would sit with their hands in their pants if there wasn't such a big taboo about doing so. But most of us suppress this type of inappropriate impulse long before we become aware of it. This pattern in our impulse control is perceived as part of our personality. In Benny's case, his dementia is affecting his personality and impulse control. Maybe to the extent that he doesn't even realise that he has his hand in his pants. That is why he is confused when Christina pulls his hand away.

If Christina thinks that Benny will learn anything from her actions, then she hasn't understood what dementia is. Furthermore, the way in which she expresses herself implies that she thinks it is Benny's responsibility not to sit with his hand in his pants. Christina's way of handling the situation will probably have the result that Benny will sit many more times with his hand in his pants and that Christina will become more and more irritated with him. And as for Benny, he will probably be more and more miserable and more and more unsure of the staff.

Christina's belief that Benny will learn from the situation means that she is trying to solve two problems at the same time. First, that Benny is sitting right now with his hand in his pants. Second, that he might sit with his hand there in the future too. But you can't solve two problems with one solution. Usually two solutions are needed. It would therefore have been a good idea for Christina to first solve the problem she had in front of her, and, later on, to try and develop a solution for the future. This means that she needs to introduce a method called distraction.

DISTRACTION AS A METHOD

The value of distraction as a method is underestimated. Everyone who works with people uses distractions, and, in private life, we distract each other and our children all the time. The advantage of distraction is that it is a here-and-now method, which transforms a situation without causing conflict. And that is worth a lot. If Christina instead of setting a limit had said: 'Look Benny, there are pictures of cars in the paper. Was it one of those you had?' then Benny probably would have taken his hand out of his pants and looked at the paper with her. Because he has been interested in cars all his life.

Distractions solve a problem here and now. But it doesn't prevent the same problem from arising again in the future. The idea that an intervention here and now can solve a problem in the future is based on the concept of learning. And that is absurd when it comes to people with dementia. Benny learnt ages ago that you're not meant to sit with your hand in your pants in public situations. He just can't stop himself from doing it any longer.

We have an important principle here. We cannot solve a situation here and now and at the same time prevent it from happening again. We need to apply a model of situation management and change that reads:

1. Manage the situation without escalating the situation.

2. Evaluate. What went wrong?

3. Change what needs to be changed in order to avoid repeating the situation next time.

WE NEED A PLAN

In order to solve a problem that arises, and that may arise again in the future, we need to know how we should act in a good way right now. But we also need to plan how we will act when, in spite of everything, it happens again, as it surely will.

In the days of mental hospitals, many people with dementia wore pants that they couldn't put their hands into. This was obviously a simple but rather inhuman method called mechanical fixation. It belongs in the same category as straitjackets and belts, which of course deprive a person of his personality. It is part of being human to be able to put your hand inside your pants if you want to. If we reintroduced that type of method, it wouldn't take very long before we accepted other limit-setting methods as well, such as locking people up, strapping them in bed, and so on. So that is something we definitely don't recommend.

So if Christina and her colleagues are to make a plan that will ensure that Benny doesn't put his hands in his pants again, it must involve keeping him busy with activities that make sense and require him to use both hands. But it is important that the activity makes sense for him, not that it makes sense for the staff. But Benny is an old man who has great contentment from doing nothing some of the time. So it will probably be hard to keep him entirely away from situations where he puts his hand in his pants. Therefore a plan is also needed for what Christina and her colleagues should do when he in fact does this.

A good action plan is to have a whole load of distractions up your sleeve. Every time Benny sits in a communal area, the staff should keep an eye on him. Then if he crosses the border for what they think is acceptable behaviour, they should use a distraction. This doesn't mean that they should distract him every time he sits close to a woman. But if they notice that the woman is unhappy with Benny's behaviour, then it's time for a distraction. So it's a good idea to have a list of possible distractions for older people who might need them, and to ensure that all staff members are aware of them. We will look more at distractions and action plans in the second part of the book.

Summary
Many of our methods build on people being able to learn from them. But since people with dementia no longer learn, we need to become aware about which of our methods depend on people being able to learn. Because those we shouldn't use. Methods that focus on preventing and managing behaviour that challenges are usually better.

6

You Need Self-control to Cooperate with Others

NANCY

Nancy doesn't want to get up and wash herself in the morning. She scolds the staff when they come in to wake her. If they take hold of her blanket she spits and claws at them. The situation around her morning ablutions has escalated more and more, and in the view of the staff the problem is aggravated by the fact that Nancy almost always wets her bed. This means that if they let Nancy stay in bed until she wakes up on her own, she'll put something dry on top of the wet clothes and refuse to change into anything else for the rest of the day. Which means that she walks about in clothes that smell strongly of urine and that she greatly disturbs the other residents, who complain loudly about the smell.

One morning Nancy has wet her bed as usual. Fatima is a new employee who goes into Nancy's room. She sits down on the floor near the top of the bed and says quietly: 'Good morning, would you like to get up now?' Nancy opens her eyes briefly and says: 'Go away, leave me alone.' Fatima waits ten minutes and then sits down again in the same way and says, 'Good morning, would you like to get up now?' Nancy opens her eyes, looks at Fatima and says: 'I'm sleeping', and then closes her eyes again. Fatima leaves and comes back in the same way after ten more minutes. Before Fatima has a chance to say anything, Nancy opens her eyes and says: 'I'm going to pee.' Fatima answers: 'Shall we go together?' And they go to the bathroom. Since Nancy's clothes are wet with urine, she says while sitting on the toilet: 'Yuck, how cold it is here.' 'Would you perhaps like to take a lovely warm bath?' Fatima asks. Yes, Nancy would like that very much.

IT DOESN'T HELP TO REPRIMAND
PEOPLE WHO ARE IN AFFECT

The principle 'You need self-control to cooperate with others' is simple. We often think that we can tell people who are stressed and agitated to calm down and that they will then do so. But that is not the case. A person in affect is a person who can't think normally and who reacts on impulse to a higher degree than usual. Neither will raising one's voice in such a situation have the desired effect.

If we look at the situation with Nancy in light of the principles discussed earlier, we see that she is unable to control her anger when the staff take hold of her blanket. She does what is most understandable in the situation from her agitated perspective – she scratches and spits.

As staff, there are many situations where we have to handle anger and lack of self-control from older people. Sometimes by saving a situation here and now, and sometimes by just waiting in the background, like Fatima does in the situation described above. The important thing, however, is that we are aware of what is really happening in situations that arise because someone has a behaviour problem, and that we know how to act in the various phases of the situation. In 1983, researchers Stephen G. Kaplan and Eugenie G. Wheeler made a basic model for an outburst of affect, which has since been presented in countless versions. Here is our version, developed by one of the book's co-authors, Bo Hejlskov Elvén:

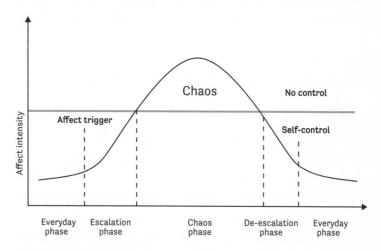

Figure 6.1 The affect regulation model

The vertical axis shows the intensity of affect, that is to say the strength of the emotion, and from left to right we have time. The curve describes the development of affect in a conflict or chaos situation, and the horizontal line in the centre shows how much affect a person can take. Newborn babies can't take very much, they lose control every time they get hungry, so for them the line would be very low. With increasing age, tolerance for affect increases, and in our model this means that the line for a child will rise. This is called maturing. As adults we can handle most situations. So in the model, the line for most of us would lie above the curve. As we age and lose abilities and cognitive functions, however, the line begins to fall again. In dementia, the line is often as low as for a little child. This is called having *difficulty in regulating affect*. Most people who lose their self-control become unhappy; some react with anger. So it is throughout life.

There are five areas in the model, which describe different phases of an outburst. In the first phase, the everyday phase, affect intensity is low. In Nancy's case, this is when she is having a good day in which everything is as it should be and she feels secure. Then comes a trigger factor, an affect trigger. For Nancy, this occurs when the staff wake her up. During this phase, the escalation phase, the staff can still communicate with her. Admittedly communication is not as good as in the everyday phase, but there is still a chance of resolving the situation. And since no-one wants to lose control, everyone usually tries to resolve the situation in this phase. For Nancy, this takes the form of scolding the staff. This is an attempt at resolving the situation from her side.

Sometimes the situation moves on into the chaos phase. This could have happened with Nancy if the staff had carried on pulling at her blanket in spite of her warning cries. In the chaos phase, the person in affect is beyond reach and no longer acts strategically. After a while, however (because it always passes), the person gradually calms down and eventually comes back to the everyday phase.

Everyone behaves differently in the different phases. To be able to resolve a situation like the one with Nancy in a good way, we need to use different methods in the different phases. We will go through this in the coming chapters and also in the second part of the book.

But it is important to highlight here that cooperation is only possible when a person lies under the line that shows how much affect the person can tolerate. If the intensity of affect rises above the line, then there is no possibility for communication at all.

We get the best cooperation in the everyday phase, when a person has full self-control. In the escalation and de-escalation phases, cooperation is more difficult but still possible. It will require more adjustment on our part if we are to succeed here, however, because in these phases the person is fully occupied with himself and his efforts to maintain control.

In order to always be able to recognise what phase of affect a person is in, we should make efforts to get to know them as well as possible. We also need to know something about possible affect triggers for that person (things we absolutely must not say or do) and what we can do in each phase so that the intensity of affect will fall and the person will regain their self-control and the ability to cooperate. In Nancy's case, Fatima's approach worked as a slow but careful method which got her to cooperate, but which still allowed Nancy to retain the initiative. Fatima followed Nancy instead of placing demands. By physically withdrawing several times, she kept Nancy's affect level below the line. In this way she encouraged, 'snoozed' and prepared Nancy for what was going to happen. This allowed Nancy to accept Fatima's suggestions on her own terms.

Summary
Cooperation is about two people adjusting their behaviour to each other. This requires that both of them have control over themselves. As staff working with a person with dementia, we therefore cannot take control. We must instead make sure that the person has control over himself.

7

Everyone Does What They Can to Maintain Self-control

RALPH

Ralph is wandering back and forth in the corridor and the staff see that he has excrement running out of his trouser leg as he walks. Since Ralph is not the easiest person to help, the staff decide that both Sue and Betty should help him. Sue leads Ralph into the bathroom and Betty goes to fetch clean clothes.

While Sue is undressing Ralph, Betty comes back with the clean clothes. Ralph looks up in fright and exclaims: 'What does she want?' Betty answers: 'I'm here to help you because you have poo everywhere.' Ralph gets very angry and looks at Sue. He looks at her with a very special, staring and mean look. Ralph shoves her away and shouts: 'I don't want help. Get out, both of you!'

Sue and Betty call for more help and Pablo and Camilla arrive. Three of them hold Ralph while Sue washes him. He bites, spits and head-butts while shouting: 'Assault, assault! Call the police!' Finally they can't hold him any longer, and before getting any clothes on he runs trouser-less out into the corridor, knocking over everything he can reach. After a few minutes he sits down on a chair and just stares into space.

NO-ONE WANTS TO LOSE CONTROL

The principle 'Everyone does what they can to maintain self-control' is also one that most of us can relate to from our own lives. We humans simply do everything we can in order not to lose control. This is not so strange. None of us want to throw furniture around, break windows, shout, fight or butt our head against the wall. So we do what we can to avoid ending up in chaos, especially when we are in the escalation phase of the model described in the previous chapter. Some of our methods are effective and good:

- Trying to withdraw from difficult situations in order to get a little peace and quiet.

- Screening yourself off, so that you can remain in the situation without the difficult part being so difficult.

- Deciding that things are going to be OK, and concentrating on that.

- Doing something familiar in order to feel secure. This is something we see when people with dementia try to go home to their children, or to go to work, because these are things they are used to doing.

- Looking to others for support. Either actively or just by asking questions about anything at all, in order to make contact.

At other times we use methods which are no doubt effective, but which may not be as well received by those around us:

- Refusing to participate. Just saying 'no'. This is perhaps the easiest method, but also the most dangerous. Very many conflicts between staff and a person with dementia begin with a demand that the person with dementia refuses.

- Lying in order to deal with a difficult situation. Canadian researcher Victoria Talwar has shown that we lie to protect ourselves if that is the easiest way out. Normal adults usually lie in a sophisticated way, so that it is not detected, but it is easy to tell when someone is lying badly. To lie well you have to be good at calculating how other people think, feel and perceive things. Unfortunately these are skills that are often affected by the development of dementia. This means that we have to take this lack of competence into account for older people who we think lie a lot. They are doing their best, but not succeeding very well. So as professionals, we shouldn't be irritated with people who lie. The reason we get irritated is that they lie so badly that it is obvious they are lying. If they were better at lying, we would not have noticed. But we work with people with dementia because they are not very good at things any more. It's part of the package, so to speak.

- Threatening to leave or to hit someone.

- Running away.

- Hitting out at others so that they will keep their distance.

- Seeking social acceptance by using insults and the like.

The methods in the second list could be perceived as behaviour that challenges. It is therefore important to be aware that these are strategic behaviours that a person with dementia resorts to in order to resolve a situation, not to spoil it. This means that we have to try to avoid placing a moral filter on the behaviour. The behaviour in itself is not wrong, and the alternative would presumably have been even worse. So if we want to change a certain behaviour we must go back to the principles and find out why the behaviour arises in the first place. Then we can change the circumstances so that it doesn't happen again.

It is useless to talk to a person with dementia about what he has done wrong. Because this assumes that he is able to learn and remember for the next time. Ralph in the example above does what seems best to him in the situation. Each time. Even when it involves shouting and crying and running out into the corridor without pants. If we look back at the affect-regulation model, we can see that all methods used during the escalation phase must have as their final objective to help the person maintain his self-control. Not that we take control, as the staff tried to do with Ralph by holding him. Because that doesn't work. Ralph can only cooperate if he has control over himself. In the same way, Nancy can only cooperate if she feels that she has control over herself and her situation when it's time to get up in the morning.

Summary

As humans, we always try to maintain our self-control. Sometimes with good methods, but often with methods that could be perceived as behaviour that challenges. For example, perhaps we lie in order to handle a difficult situation, or we leave when things get uncomfortable. People with dementia do the same.

8

Affect Is Contagious

BERTHA AND SEYMOUR

It's afternoon and there is a pleasant atmosphere in the care home. A couple of members of staff are moving around serving coffee to the residents, who are sitting in small groups, drinking coffee and watching TV. One resident, Bertha, is sitting with a dementia doll, talking to it now and then, while Seymour is sitting staring into space. The municipality's supervisor for dementia care comes by and says that she will be around for the next few hours, to observe the daily life of the residents.

Nursing assistant Louise, who is in the kitchen, hasn't heard about this and calls out into the corridor to her colleague Sophie: 'Sophie, did you know we were getting a visitor today?' Sophie answers, but Louise can't hear her and so she calls again, louder, repeating the question. It's a bit noisy in the background, partly because of a janitor who is fixing a lamp, and partly because of the TV. In the midst of all this, another member of staff is on her way home. She waves to her colleagues and says: 'Bye, have a nice shift!'

The effect on the residents of all these sounds and disturbances in the room is that they start to get up, walk around anxiously, and look for the staff. They become what we often call appellant. Bertha, who earlier on was entertaining herself with the dementia doll looks up and says: 'Hello, hello, do I have to be here?' While Seymour goes out into the kitchen and asks: 'What should I do now?' A minute later a third person, Eugene, gets up decisively and says: 'OK, I'm off to work now. Bye!' He goes over to the door and on outside while the staff have their hands full with the others. They don't discover that Eugene has left until half an hour later when things have settled down again.

AFFECT CONTAGION AND THE BRAIN

The principle 'Affect is contagious' was formulated by psychologist Silvan Tomkins in the 1960s. He based his thinking on observations made by researchers in psychology as early as the 1880s. Later, in the 1990s, Italian Giacomo Rizzolatti discovered how the process works. He found that the pattern of activity in a person's brain when he does something is mirrored in other people's brains. This means that if the person smiles, then all those who see that smile will have the same pattern of activity in their brains as if they had been the one who smiled. Which may lead to them actually smiling back. Rizzolatti calls this 'mirror neuron processes'.

As humans, we perceive other people's feelings by being infected by them. It is thus easier to be happy if we are together with happy people, and we grow calmer when we are with calm people. But there is variation in how easily we are infected by other people's feelings. Some of us are influenced very little by other people's feelings, others are somewhat affected by how people around us are feeling, and still others are completely at the mercy of other people's feelings.

In a care home we are likely to find all types, which means that the general atmosphere will be influenced by the mood of both the residents and the members of staff. But it also means that some people with dementia will be strongly affected if the staff set boundaries and scold. Their reaction will be to start scolding as well. Just by their personality and manner, such staff create strong anxiety in older people. This doesn't necessarily have to be a problem, but it may mean that this type of person should not work with the most affect-sensitive people in the home.

If we look at the example above and go back to the principles in the first chapter, we can conclude that the staff in the coffee-time situation are asking too much of the older people's ability to regulate affect. Just the fact that they shout to each other makes Bertha and the others start activating strategies for maintaining control (seeking support from the staff, wanting to go to work). The staff are responsible for the unease that arises. They have to change their behaviour.

The more conflicts we have with a person the more important this is. When we have a lot of conflicts with someone, a very normal reaction is for us to become more decisive in our tone of voice and our body language. Unfortunately, this has the result that the other person also becomes more decisive, increasing the risk of conflict. We perhaps then react by using marked body language. Perhaps we demand eye contact. And perhaps we move closer to the other person in the demand situation. But all these behaviours increase the transmission of affect to the other person and thereby the risk of conflict.

To avoid such a situation, reduce the risk of conflict, and instead increase the possibility of a good resolution, the following are important:

- *Never demand eye contact.* This is a simple domination tool that most often results in escalation of a conflict.

- *Never maintain eye contact for longer than you would have done in a calm situation.* Prolonged eye contact increases the transmission of affect.

- *Take a step away, or walk backwards, in a potential conflict situation.* By going closer when we are making a demand or setting a boundary, we greatly increase the person's stress level.

- *Take a step back at the same time as you make a demand.* Then the stress of the demand will be balanced by reduced affect transmission.

- *Sit down when the person is uneasy, or lean against a wall.* A calm body is just as infectious as a tense one, but infects with calm. And we want the person to be calm.

- *Distract rather than confront.* By changing the person's focus we take away the affect transmission that arises between us in situations where we want to set a boundary. We distract by getting the person to think about something else. In the escalation phase of the model described in the Chapter 6, distraction is probably the most important active method to use.

- *Refrain from taking hold of the person with tensed muscles.* Muscle tension is infectious just like affect is. This means that if the person takes hold of us, we must try to relax in order to get the person to let go. This is the opposite of our first impulse, but not so difficult when you think about it.

- *If we must take hold of someone, do it calmly and move with the person's movements, not against them.* And only for a few seconds at a time, then let go. In that short time the person has time to become distracted, and when we let go the person usually regains their self-control. To physically restrain a person by holding them tightly will in most cases result in violent conflict.

There is another little principle that perhaps should really have a chapter of its own but which we will only touch on briefly here: 'The one who wins loses'. If we win a conflict with a person who has dementia, it will not improve the person's quality of life or tendency to cooperate. But since we actually don't want anyone to lose, this also means that no-one can win. Instead of getting into a relationship of opposition with the person, we need to get them to go in the same direction as us. Methods that are based on dominance have a different objective and rarely help us reach the goals we have in dementia and older care.

Summary

Affect is contagious. If we are together with happy people we become happier than if we are together with people who are depressed. We therefore have to be aware of both our own feelings and the feelings of older people. By using active strategies to reduce affect in them we can also prevent and manage behaviour that challenges.

9

Conflicts Consist of Solutions *and* Failures Require an Action Plan

IRMA

Irma often goes in to the other residents' rooms in the care home and when the staff follow her, she feels pursued. She then tries to grab a few small items from the room and runs away to hide them. Several residents have complained, and two relatives have also complained that Irma goes into their relatives' rooms. At a meeting it is decided that Irma should have a fixed guard to keep an eye on her, so that she doesn't go into the others' rooms. From the very first day with her guard, Ross, Irma tries to run away from him. Before the week is over she has managed to evade him twice and go outside, and the police have had to drive her back to the care home on both occasions. On a third occasion Ross finds her before she has got that far, but since she hits him and scratches him in the face when he tries to bring her back to the care home, he is forced to take hold of her. It takes a long time for Irma to calm down after getting back to her room.

CONFLICTS CONSIST OF SOLUTIONS

The principle 'Conflicts consist of solutions' is not difficult to understand either. If we look at Irma's and Ross's behaviour, one action at a time, we will see that the situation develops according to a simple pattern. One person has a problem. He solves the problem, but usually in a way that makes a problem for someone else. This person in turn solves the problem in his way, making a new problem for the first person to solve. That solution too becomes a problem for the other person. In this way the situation develops through a pattern of solutions that all create problems for the other party. And as the solutions multiply, so the level of violence increases, finally reaching physical conflict.

In the example above, Irma herself doesn't have a problem to begin with; she is amusing herself by going into other people's rooms and looking at their things. But the staff have a problem with her behaviour and their solution is to stay close to her and to follow her around. But this solution becomes a problem for Irma, who tries to solve it by taking things with her as she leaves the rooms. She runs away with the items and hides them so that she can look at them later. This is considered a problem by the staff. And so the escalation has begun. The staff solve the problem with a guard. Irma sees the guard as a problem and solves it by running away. The staff see the running away as a problem, which Ross solves by bringing Irma back, using force to avoid being scratched in the face. The conflict has now turned physical.

This type of conflict can only be solved by one party finding a solution that is not a problem for the other party. And here comes the most interesting part. In most such cases that we have come across in our work, we have been asked how we can teach the older person in question to find solutions to his problem that are not a problem for the staff.

But it is we, being staff, who are the professionals. We are the ones with responsibility for the everyday life and for the well-being and development of the residents. How in the world, then, can we arrive at the conclusion that it is the older person who should solve the problem? It is much simpler for us to find a solution that doesn't create problems for him.

In many of the situations in this book, the staff think they have to win. They also think they have the right to make decisions and dominate the situation. In their opinion it is the residents with dementia, like Nancy, Ralph and Irma, who must change their behaviour. All these assumptions remove the staff's ability to make a difference – for the simple reason that they carry with them the certainty of failure. Because the risk of failure when we use this type of thinking is very high. So we have to find solutions that are less risky.

A good solution must build on the idea that, as staff, we do not create problems for people with dementia. Irma solves her own problems. She has no intention of losing. The staff's escalation means that in the end they are forced into using physical violence, which will lead to Irma's strategies becoming still more powerful. And then the staff lose. Because their task is to create a good life for Irma, and they are not doing so in the situation described. They will also get new scratches and hits.

As professionals, we have an ongoing responsibility to consider the effects of our actions so that we can judge whether we are unintentionally creating more negative affect, bad feelings or escalation of a conflict. If so, we have to act differently and strive to find solutions that don't create problems for the older person. In Irma's case, for example, the staff could perhaps have tried to find out why she was going into other people's rooms. Then maybe they could have satisfied her need and her curiosity in a different way, by providing her with other activities that were meaningful for her, so that they had the initiative, not Irma. Presumably the staff's initiative would have been better than Irma's. But since they didn't have a good activity to offer her, she had one for them.

This leads us to the next principle: 'Failures require an action plan'. The principle was formulated against the background of Matthew Goodman's death. Matthew was a 14-year-old boy with extensive special education needs. He attended a special school where he fell because his arms and legs were mechanically immobilised with splints. Due to the fall he was unable to breathe, and died. In the opinion of the court, use of physical restraints by the school to limit a person's freedom of movement was a pedagogical failure, because it meant that they had not succeeded with other methods. In this case the school's failure resulted in Matthew's death. So Matthew's Law was formulated: 'All restraints are a failure. All pedagogical failures require an action plan.'

Setting Ross as a guard to keep an eye on Irma becomes a problem if his assignment is to stop her physically when she wants to go away. It only means that if Ross is violent then she will react even more violently. Already the first time he stops her and she scratches him, a pedagogical failure has taken place. An action plan is needed.

In the chaos phase in particular, it is important not to limit a person's freedom of movement. If we carry away or hold the person still in this phase, we will considerably extend its duration. To hold onto someone with tense muscles furthermore has the effect that muscle tension increases, and thereby also the stress level, adrenaline rush and risk of violence. If absolutely necessary, we can take hold of a person to avoid immediate danger to life and health. This is considered an emergency measure under the criminal code in most countries and is therefore legal. But just because it's legal doesn't mean that it's effective in the long run.

Emergency measures, by definition, should only be used in an emergency. Emergencies are rare and unpredictable occurrences. We have sometimes met staff who tell us that they regularly hold down a person when he acts out. This can never be considered an emergency measure. If a person is violent at regular intervals, then it is not unpredictable. Then as staff we instead have to think about the demands and expectations we are placing on the person in the situations where this happens, so that we can avoid them.

This means that we can employ emergency measures once or twice when a new situation arises. But the third time it happens it has become a method, and then it is not an emergency any more. So we can't drag people back to their care home while they scratch and fight. Instead we have to adjust the circumstances to prevent such things happening again, and we have to make a plan for how we will act if they still do happen. All pedagogical failures require an action plan.

Summary
It takes two to fight. This means that every conflict has two parties, both of whom are trying to solve a problem. If as staff we can adapt our problem solving to the unequal situation that exists in older and dementia care, taking into account both differing individual abilities and our own formal role, then we will be able to avoid many conflicts.

10

Pedagogy and Care Involve Making the Right Demands in a Way that Works

PETER

Aischa is sitting in the office when Peter, a man in a wheelchair, rolls in. He is very upset and shouts: 'Call the police. Call the police! I'm being pursued!' And this is admittedly true since Adam, one of the staff, is right behind him and wants to keep him from wheeling into the office. But the more Adam tries to persuade Peter to go with him, the more upset Peter gets.

Aischa thinks that Peter will calm down if someone listens to him, so she takes him at his word and makes as if to call the police. But first she asks Peter for a little more information. She takes pen and paper to make notes and asks him to tell her more. 'What has happened that I need to call the police for?' she asks. 'They follow me around and tell me that I live here! And I'm not allowed to decide for myself what I'm going to eat either. And he's part of it!' Peter points accusingly at Adam who backs away a little. 'OK, so that's how it is. I'll just write it down.' She reads out loud while writing: 'They decide...' Peter carries on explaining. 'Yes, and imagine, there I was standing just the other day, quietly eating ice-cream with my kids, and there they were again, wanting me to...'

Peter goes on describing other occasions when he has felt unfairly treated and, while he is talking, he gets more and more angry. So Aischa tries to divert his thoughts from his perceived wrongs through various distractions: 'You know, my throat is completely parched from all this talking. Wouldn't you like to have a glass of water while we carry on talking?' She fetches a glass of water and they drink a little before going on with the conversation. She moves on to the next distraction: 'Really! Here we are sitting together chatting and I didn't even get around to greet you properly.' Aischa puts out her hand and introduces herself and Peter tells her his name.

Once Peter has described all the various incidents he is no longer so hysterical but goes on with his story more quietly, describing among other things how he is not allowed to call his fiancée. Since this is a wish that Aischa can grant, they immediately place a call to his wife and Peter tells her: 'I've had such a terrible day, but luckily now I'm sitting and chatting with my lawyer, and she's really good.' After talking on the phone for a while, Peter ends the conversation and he is now glad that he has accomplished what he intended to. He ends by asking if he might not have the 'lawyer's' business card, which of course she gives him, and he walks happily away.

GUNLAYA

Gunlaya has progressed far into her dementia. She has lost all language skills and finds it very difficult to understand her environment. This brings major problems for the staff when trying to get her to cooperate in her personal hygiene. Tooth brushing is especially difficult and every time they end up with several of the staff holding her while they brush her teeth.

The staff have tried to solve this problem in different ways. They have tried to brush her teeth in different places in her room, in the communal areas, and at different times of day. They have studied her life history (she grew up in Thailand) and tried to find a Thai toothbrush in the hopes that she will recognise it. But none of these attempts have made the tooth brushing any easier, and so the physical restraint continues. The staff are no longer bothered by it, however; they see the use of force as unavoidable and it has become part of Gunlaya's and their everyday life, since she is unable to cooperate.

The problem only disappears when, during an inspection by the overseeing authorities, the staff are asked about Gunlaya's best remaining functions. They reply that she has lost practically all her functions, but that surprisingly enough she still manages to feed herself, even using a knife and fork. This gives the staff the idea of exchanging the fork for a toothbrush at the end of the evening meal to see what will happen if Gunlaya – by mistake the first time – puts the toothbrush into her mouth. The idea is a success – the very first time they try it Gunlaya brushes her teeth herself. So this becomes a regular routine and there is no longer any need for the staff to use force.

DEMANDS AS A PEDAGOGICAL TOOL

The first part of this principle, 'Pedagogy and care involve making the right demands', is easy to relate to. If it weren't true, there would be no need for schools, universities or care homes. All pedagogical work is about getting people to do things they wouldn't have done if they hadn't been part of a context. This of course also applies to care of older people. Older people receive support in their own homes or a place in a care home because they no longer can do what they used to do. Otherwise it would be enough for them to receive practical help in the form of cooking and cleaning.

Philosopher Martha Nussbaum says that all pedagogical work and all work in care is based to some degree on taking away the basic right to self-determination. This is an interesting perspective. And it is easy to understand her thinking. Because of course we don't allow people with dementia to decide entirely what they want to do, how often they shower, brush their teeth or take a walk. After all, they are in a care home because they haven't been able to manage everyday life well enough on their own. This means that as staff we have quite a heavy responsibility. Nussbaum is of the opinion that it doesn't have to be a problem in itself that we take away a person's autonomy. But we must have a good reason for doing so. Always.

The arguments that we have found in our work to be relevant in this regard are:

- *Avoidance of danger.* People with dementia illnesses should preferably be where we can keep an eye on them. This is not particularly controversial. They can easily get lost and get seriously hurt or even killed if left to go about on their own. The basic principle in Sweden, for example, is that people may not be locked up as long as there is no court order giving the right to do so, either a criminal sentence or through special laws on psychiatric care. It is understandable that, to avoid danger, we still make it difficult for the residents in a care home to leave, for example by placing a dark mat in front of the door going outside, as described earlier in Chapter 3. This is the same argument we use when we resort to emergency measures, for example when we take hold of someone to prevent them from running straight into the traffic.

- *Care.* We use the care argument when we require good hygiene, for example. When avoiding danger, we may use some fairly far-reaching methods, bordering on domination and control. This is not possible when using the care argument. Grabbing hold of a person who is heading into the traffic would not be seen as excessive, but brushing someone's teeth with force, as in Gunlaya's case, is definitely crossing the line in many people's view. On the other hand, we can use various tricks and even some manipulation when invoking the care argument. For example, allowing ourselves to add swimming to a person's weekly schedule so as to ensure that they shower at least once a week.

- *Increasing actual autonomy.* This is the ultimate argument. Many people with dementia can't handle full self-determination. Neither can normal people. Society has followed the implications of this by limiting our autonomy on certain points. A good example is traffic. The lawmakers have decided that we may only drive on one side of the road. This can be seen as a serious restriction of normal people's autonomy. At the same time, it means that our ability to go wherever we want increases considerably. Because if we had been allowed to drive on either side of the road we wouldn't have been able to get very far. Similarly, many people with dementia wouldn't be able to do very much on their own and would become quite apathetic if the initiative was left entirely up to them. Many would soon die of hunger if they weren't offered food. That is why we offer activities and serve food, so that they can make choices. But every time we say that it's time to eat, we are actually limiting their freedom of choice.

One of the principles we have already discussed is 'People always do what makes sense' (see Chapter 3). This implies that if we choose to guide a person's behaviour in a certain direction (because we have a good reason for doing so), then we can get help from the concept of making sense. This can be done in different ways. The simplest is to offer understandable structures. This we explained when we considered rules as well as physical and time-related structures for creating predictability. These methods are basic to all good pedagogy and care. If we have good and understandable rules to relate to, and if the physical and time-related frameworks create good behaviour and a predictable daily routine, then we have come far. For people with dementia, some activities don't make sense regardless of what we do. If these activities are important, then we must find ways to make them understandable in the situation in question. We must provide meaning. We can do this in various ways:

- *Increase the sense of involvement.* If a person with dementia feels that he has taken part in selecting an activity, then it is easier for him to participate. This doesn't mean that he needs to decide about all activities or plan them on a high, overall level. Sometimes it's enough to be involved in the small things. For example by saying: 'Do you want this towel or that one, now that you're going to have a shower?'

- *Create a sense of belonging.* If a person with dementia feels that he is seen by the staff, his confidence and trust will increase. This is often enough to create meaningfulness around following directions and meeting demands. It still means that we have to ensure that the demands we make are not too high. If they are, trust will diminish and behaviour that challenges increase. In older care, the 'we-method' has received a bad reputation. Saying, for example: 'Shall we go to the toilet?' Of course we shouldn't say that we also are going to the toilet when we don't actually intend to do so. On the other hand, it is perfectly OK to use the we-method for activities that we ourselves participate in. Because it is easier to do something if one is doing it together with other people. The toilet situation itself is interesting in several ways. If we say 'You must go and pee' because we don't want to use the we-method, then we diminish the sense of autonomy. The person with dementia may not think that this is something someone else should be deciding for him. A better method would be to say: 'Shall we see if we can find a toilet so that you can have a pee?'

- *Create predictability.* The better prepared a person with dementia is, the easier it will be for him to participate. So it is important to say what is going to happen shortly before an activity begins, as long as the person is able to remember it for a minute or two. It is also good to announce when there are only a few minutes of an activity left, to prepare the person that it will soon be over. It is best, however, for the activities in a care home to follow a pattern that is familiar to the residents; things that they have done many times in their lives.

- *Increase meaningfulness through out-and-out tricks.* One example can be to make use of the word 'done'. When an activity is done, it is natural to begin something new. Some activities have a clear 'done', like when you eat. So if we prepare for a new activity by saying 'When you are done eating, we are going to...', then most people will be able to stop what they are doing and move on. 'Done' also works in group situations. For example, if you are on a field trip and want everyone to be ready to leave for the trip home, you can offer them an ice-cream or a banana. Then everyone interrupts whatever they are doing in order to eat. When that activity is done, everyone will be ready to go home. Yet another trick is to count to three, a quick and recognisable way to prepare people that something is going to happen. A classic pedagogical method is to use a prompt. For example, if we give a person a towel, it becomes easier for him to take a shower. This method is good for things of a more challenging nature, such as we saw in the example of Gunlaya. The use of more than one prompt at the same time is very effective, such as prompting for a meal by setting the table, letting the aroma of cooking spread and saying 'Lunchtime!' Then everyone knows what is about to happen. This is a great help for people who have difficulty orienting themselves because of dementia.

- *Use motivating activities.* This could mean adding a competitive element to a boring activity or putting fun into situations that could potentially become chaotic. Simply making an activity more exciting by adding something interesting or fun.

Making demands might be about getting a person with dementia to eat or take a shower. But it could also be about getting a person to take his hands out of his pants or persuading someone to stay out of other people's rooms. We have already discussed setting boundaries, but let's consider this again. We must differentiate between demands that are about what we want someone to do and what we want them to stop doing.

If a person is already engaged in a behaviour that we need to interrupt, the demand we try to make is often very clear and reprimanding in nature. As we have already seen, there is unfortunately nothing to suggest that we can bring about long-term changes in behaviour by setting boundaries. At best, boundary-setting, then, is only a way to handle an immediate, difficult situation. At the same time it is a risky way. Norwegian research, for example, has shown that violence against staff often arises out of situations where the staff are trying to set a boundary. But it doesn't change anything in the long run. Rather, it risks creating a conflict situation. Then distraction is a better alternative. With the help of distractions we can change the focus by talking about things that interest the person, catch his attention, or get him to think about something else. Once again – not everyone needs this type of intervention. But for those who do need it, distractions can considerably reduce conflict.

Summary

Pedagogy and care are about getting people to cooperate and to do things they otherwise would not have done. When working with people that have dementia, this means that it is not enough to only make demands of them. We have not succeeded in our work until we can get them to do what is good for them. That is what we are paid to do.

11

To Lead Is to Cooperate

DONALD

Donald wanders back and forth in the corridor, like a lion in a cage, with a restless, stressed and frustrated body language. The other residents are sitting together with the staff in the lounge. There is a pleasant atmosphere in the room, and they are singing and drinking coffee. Donald, however, doesn't feel this is meaningful and he becomes more and more stressed and confrontational, and almost threatening towards those he meets in the corridor, who clearly seem afraid of him. Donald shouts: 'Now I've been at this job for ten days and still no-one has told me what I'm meant to do!' And a few minutes later: 'You're not doing a damn thing, just sitting around drinking coffee.'

One of the staff, Prue, notices that Donald is not very happy and tries a few different diversions, among them asking him: 'Donald, wouldn't you like a cup of coffee with the others?' And again a little later: 'Have you noticed that we have a new TV in the lounge? Would you like to come with us and watch TV?' Then Donald gets even angrier: 'Do you really think I want to drink coffee, we bloomin' well haven't done anything else all day. I damn well couldn't care less about your new TV!'

Then Prue's colleague, Brenda, tries a different strategy (validation, a key concept in person-centred care) by taking Donald more seriously. She asks: 'Is it true that you haven't been given any work yet?' Donald answers vehemently: 'Yes! And I've been here for two weeks!' Brenda continues: 'Really? What would you like to do if it was your choice?' Donald answers: 'Maybe a workshop where I could work a bit with some tools.' Brenda latches on to this: 'Maybe some woodworking?' At this point the conversation derails somewhat. Donald looks at Brenda confused. She tries to get back on track by using one of Donald's own words: 'You were thinking of something to do with tools?' 'Yes! I'm an old toolmaker, after all,' he replies.

Brenda and Donald then get into a long conversation about what Donald has done in the past, where he has worked and the various things he has accomplished during his career. The longer they talk about things that are important to Donald, the calmer he gets. After they have chatted for maybe 3–4 minutes, he ends the conversation himself, and stands there thinking for a while before saying: 'Well then, I'll give them two more weeks. If they haven't come up with anything by then, then I can't be bothered any more. I'll retire.' Brenda answers: 'Oh, that sounds exciting. What will you do when you retire?' 'Oh I don't know, I'll probably think of something.' Then Donald strolls quietly back and forth in the corridor, looks around, stops a minute and rocks back and forth on his feet.

TO LEAD

The principle 'To lead is to cooperate' may seem contradictory. But in dementia care in particular, it is an absolutely central concept. Because it isn't certain that the one to be led understands that he is to be led. And in other cases, older people expect leadership from us of a kind that we are not offering. So it isn't all that easy.

The above situation is really amazing. Donald is expecting that someone should make decisions for him. A boss, who should tell him what his work assignments are. Only no-one does. At least not in the way that he expects, although naturally there are aspects of both steering and authoritativeness in what the staff do.

If the staff in a situation like this had set a boundary, the situation would probably have gone out of control. Donald expects to have someone deciding for him, but only for things that he wants them to decide. The staff are welcome to tell him what to do in the workshop. But no-one is going to tell him when to drink coffee. That's something he decides for himself. Here is the core of leadership in older care. It's all about the expectations of older people.

This is actually the case everywhere, but it is especially apparent in older care because many older people have a picture of themselves and their situation that is influenced by perceptions that may not conform to reality. They live in a different time. A time when they were capable of deciding for themselves. This means that we must be extremely careful about exercising authority. But it doesn't mean that we should not lead. That is part of our job. But we have to do it in such a way that the older person feels involved.

HOBBES AND RAWLS

Leading is difficult. Research into leadership has focused to a great extent on leading businesses, which is naturally very different to leading in older and dementia care. But we can learn from the key thinkers. One of these was the British 17th-century philosopher Hobbes. He advocated a type of government that we today would describe as a dictatorship. He proposed that in exchange for their needs for security, rights and welfare being fulfilled, people would yield their freedom to a leader. If the leader then failed to provide for the people's needs, they would take back their freedom. We have seen many examples of this phenomenon, not least in Eastern Europe around 1990, and more recently in connection with the Arab Spring. The same thing happens in democracies, but democratically, through free elections.

Hobbes' principles are certainly relevant in our work-life. We do what the boss says because the boss sees to it that we are paid and that we have a good work environment. In principle, the same contract exists in the interplay between us and the people we take care of. They give up their right to self-determination in exchange for well-being and support. If as staff we fail in this, they take back their self-determination, either by questioning things or by keeping away. In dementia care, however, things are a little more complicated than in other fields.

The philosopher John Rawls has described another phenomenon by means of a few principles. In the first principle, he sees the community as consisting of many people who do not make decisions for each other, but who must cooperate. We do this by behaving decently towards each other. We all live together as if we had a contract with each other that said something like this: 'If you behave, I'll behave.' As long as it works there's no problem. The problem arises when one of us does not behave in the right way. Then Rawls' second principle comes into effect: 'If you don't behave, then I lose respect for your rights.'

These principles apply throughout society. For example, we are pretty much in agreement that it's OK to drive a little faster than the speed limit. That is still acceptable behaviour. But if someone drives much too fast, then we think that person deserves to lose their driver's licence. And if we are overtaken by a Maserati doing 270 mph, then we think that the police should confiscate the car. We have now lost respect for the owner's property rights. But Rawls' principle applies only to peers. In traffic we are all equals, so there we have to behave. In society as a whole we are also equals, so there we must also behave if we want to retain our rights.

NUSSBAUM

But in some situations we are not equals. This has been described well by the philosopher Martha Nussbaum. She says, for example, that people with disabilities differ from others since they need support. This leads to an uneven power relationship that is not on equal terms. People with disabilities are dependent on others, but others are not dependent on them. This means that from the outset they have fewer rights than others.

People with dementia who live in care homes do not have the right to move about freely in the community on their own. We have taken this right away from them because they can't handle it. We have not done this through a legal process, it's just something we have decided. Often they themselves participated in making the decision, but that's something most of them have forgotten. Since people with dementia don't have the same rights as the rest of us, they don't have to behave. That's why we don't call the police if they take someone else's sweater or go into someone else's room. We expect that such things can happen.

In caring for people with dementia, we often find ourselves in situations where the people we are caring for think they are on equal terms with us. But that is not really the case. And this is particularly challenging. Sometimes we have to use our power to ensure that they brush their teeth, shower, don't wander away and so on. But not by telling them what they may or may not do. Because they think that these are things they should decide for themselves. Donald thinks it's OK for the employer to decide what he should do in the workshop. But only in the workshop. There Hobbes' leadership principles apply. For the other parts of his life, Donald thinks that Rawls' principles apply. He makes decisions for himself and other people make decisions for themselves. And we all behave. That's why Donald expects the staff to speak politely to him and to take him seriously. That is behaving. We take each other seriously. Asking him to watch TV and drink coffee all day, on the other hand, is not behaving. So he reacts against that. But when Brenda eventually validates Donald's perception of the situation, he calms down. Then he can navigate again. Then he is back in Rawls' principles.

Brenda knows, however, that the world is different. She knows that part of her job is to get Donald to relax and not get frustrated. So she has to take the leader's position and make sure that Donald feels OK. Just as Hobbes described. In spite of this, Donald doesn't just hand over his authority to Brenda. He thinks he can manage on his own.

This is the essence of what we call person-centred care. And of dementia care in general. We have to work in a way that gets older people to cooperate with us. Not by deciding for them, but rather by getting them to feel that we are deciding together. This is why dementia care is a job that requires high qualifications and therefore should be better paid than a managerial position in a regular company.

This brings us back to the concepts of *understandability* and *making sense*. People with dementia, just like everyone else, do what is most understandable in each situation. That which makes most sense. That's why we as staff need to make the desired behaviour the one that makes most sense in every situation. This leads us back to what we earlier in the book called making sense, with regard to physical boundaries, rules and activities. But it is important that it all is founded on belonging.

POWER AND FREEDOM OF SPEECH

Before we go any further, we will just discuss one last detail about power. There are situations where we are equals, for example between friends or partners. In such situations, Rawls' principles apply: 'You don't decide for me and I don't decide for you'; 'If you behave, then I'll behave'; and 'If you don't behave, then I lose respect for your rights.' But then one day perhaps your friend or partner suddenly begins to decide about something you don't want them to decide about, over your head. You protest. You do so to point out that the balance of power has shifted and that you don't accept this. After all, your relationship is one of equals. But if a protest doesn't help, you might call the other person something you don't really mean. Maybe something rude. The other person can then choose between two courses of action:

- To say: 'I'm sorry. Of course I don't decide for you.' Equality is restored.

- To say: '#%&@ yourself.' Equality is restored. You are both #%&@s.

We use invectives to challenge power, especially when we don't think the power should lie where it does. That's why it is important that, as professionals, we don't take the invective we may get personally, but rather take it as information that we need to do something differently. Perhaps the person with dementia is cursing because they feel that decisions are being made for them, and their affect is increasing to the point where it can be difficult to maintain self-control. Cursing, in other words, is something that we have to relate to from the perspective of the special circumstances of dementia care.

HOWARD

Howard is irritated. He can't find his brown pants and is running around in his underwear looking for them. At the same time, there is a strange woman in his apartment who is constantly trying to get him to put on a pair of grey sweatpants. He would never dream of wearing sweatpants.

Howard can't understand why she's in his apartment. So he asks: 'What are you doing in my apartment? And why would I put on those dreadful sweatpants? Can you go away?' But she doesn't go away. Instead she sits down in his armchair. Then he gets angry: 'You stupid woman! Leave! Or I'll throw you out.' He moves towards her threateningly.

In Howard's world, this woman in not behaving. He doesn't understand what she's doing in his apartment. And she is not going to decide which pants he is going to wear. That, of course, is something he decides for himself. He doesn't decide for her and she doesn't decide for him. Especially not in his apartment.

TORI

Tori works in the care home where Howard lives. Her job is to see to it that Howard has a good day, among other things by making sure that he wears clothes so that he can take part in communal activities. It seems to her that Howard is running around the room in confusion, rooting around in boxes, looking under the bed and throwing things on the floor. In only his underwear. When she asks him what he's looking for, he says: 'My pants.' She holds out his pants so he can put them on. The nice new pants that his daughter brought, since he has such a hard time putting on the old ones by himself. It's much easier with sweatpants.

In the middle of everything Howard stops, looks commandingly at her and tells her to leave. But she can't do that, she hasn't finished helping him yet. So she sits down. Whereupon he suddenly gets very threatening, and calls her a stupid woman. Tori flees the room. At the next staff meeting, she brings the situation up as an example of how bad the workplace environment is.

In Tori's world, Howard is not behaving. He shouldn't call her a stupid woman. Nor should he threaten her. She's only trying to help.

The problem in this situation is that in order for Tori to help Howard, he must understand that he needs help. Only then will she be able to help him. But he thinks she just wants to decide for him. And he is certainly allowed to call anyone who wants to make decisions for him a stupid woman. In Howard's world, he and Tori are equals. So they must both behave. In Tori's world, however, she has the right to decide for Howard. This means that they are not equals. And things seldom go well with two such different starting points.

This is a challenge that arises daily in care homes in all over the world. Staff should arrange things so that each older person has a good day. But they should do so in such a way that those for whom they decide don't feel that decisions are being made for them. This means it's OK for Howard to call Tori a stupid woman. If Tori wants to find a better solution, then she must take responsibility for doing so, for example by getting Howard to decide that he wants to wear the sweatpants.

HOWARD

Howard is irritated. He can't find his brown pants and is running around in his underwear looking for them. At the same time, there is a woman in his apartment, and he can't quite understand what she is doing there. She says: 'What are you looking for?' 'My pants,' Howard answers. She shows him a pair of ugly, grey sweatpants: 'Are these the ones?' 'No,' he says. 'I never wear sweatpants. I have a brown pair with creases.' 'OK,' Tori says. 'I'll help you look.' She looks around.

After they have both searched for a while she says: 'I can't find any brown pants. Can't you put these ones on, since we're going out to have coffee with the others?' At first Howard doesn't want to. After all you can't drink coffee with strangers in your pyjamas. But after they have carried on searching for a few more minutes he puts on the grey sweatpants. At least it's better to wear them than to drink coffee with strangers in your underwear.

Here Tori validates Howard's view of the situation and gets him to decide to put on the pants. She solves the problem. And her work environment remains good the whole time.

Summary

Older and dementia care are fundamentally different from all other pedagogical contexts and care situations, because people with dementia don't know that it is the staff who decide. They think that they decide for themselves. This means that we must continually get them to choose to cooperate. Which means that we can't be authoritarian. Our task is to get them to do what is good for them, and to do so in such a way that they believe they are making their own decisions.

Part 2

Cases and Action Plans

This second part of the book is about how, in concrete terms, we put the responsibility principle into practice, find the tools we need for the job and, not least, learn when to use the different tools. After all, it is our responsibility to fulfil the task that society has given us. And there are no good excuses for failure.

We will consider three situations and try to understand them in relation to the principles described in the first part of the book. With the help of the model (Figure 6.1) we looked at earlier on, we will analyse the situations and approach them in an effective way.

12

We Work in a Garage

We will begin the second part of the book by drawing up the course. This we will do using a simple metaphor: we work in a garage. Our job is to perform the tasks that society has assigned us. Service and repair of older people. Service and repairs are what we do, and for these we need good tools and methods.

When the car breaks down we usually take it to a garage. Basically, we enter into a contract with the mechanic that he will do a job and be paid for it. As car owners, we expect the mechanic to fulfil his part of the contract and he, in his turn, expects us to fulfil our part of the contract. The contract primarily defines who is responsible for what, and what the consequences will be if one of the parties doesn't live up to his responsibility. Society has entered into a similar contract with older care providers. Our job is to make sure that people with dementia have a good life and live as long as possible.

Suppose you have left your car at the garage for a routine service. The oil is to be changed and the mechanic is to check that everything is working properly. When you come back to pick up the car, the mechanic wants his money first, so you pay. But then it starts to get weird. Maybe the mechanic says:

- 'I haven't changed the oil. To change the oil, you have to unscrew the oil plug and drain the oil. And the plug was stuck. If the car doesn't want to cooperate, it can't be my responsibility to change the oil.'

- 'I haven't changed the oil. To change the oil, you have to unscrew the oil plug and drain the oil. The oil plug in your car is 5/8 inches. Unfortunately I don't have a 5/8 inch spanner. Most cars have 17 mm oil plugs, so that's the tool I have.'

- 'I haven't changed the oil. And you can't take the car. We have to wait for the police to get here. To change the oil, you have to unscrew the oil plug and drain the oil. The plug in your car is 5/8 inches. Unfortunately I don't have a 5/8 inch spanner. Most cars have 17 mm oil plugs, and so that's the tool I have. But 5/8 inches is the same as 15.875 mm, and so I used a 16 mm spanner. But when I was using it to try and loosen the plug, the spanner slipped and I hit my knuckles on the undercarriage so hard they started to bleed. Here in the garage we have zero tolerance for violence so I have reported the car to the police. So you'll have to wait until the police arrive.'

- 'We have had some downsizing here at the garage. This means that I haven't had the time to take care of your car. But it has been here and you must understand that we can't complete all assignments with the budget that we have here.'

- 'I haven't changed the oil. I don't know how it's done. But I tried for several hours and naturally I want to be paid for that.'

- 'I haven't changed the oil. When I was going to start working on the car I drove it into the garage, and while I was doing so the car started throwing its engine parts around. They were flying all over the place. Obviously I can't work under conditions like that. So I pushed it back out into the yard. You'll have to take it home. It's just in the way here. But I want to be paid in any case since I didn't have any less work to do; after all, it threw parts everywhere that I had to clean.'

- 'I haven't changed the oil. I can tell that you drive the car much too hard and then the oil gets used up faster. If you're going to drive like that, then it can't be my responsibility to change the oil more often.'

I think we can quickly agree that you are not going to go back to that garage. You expect that a mechanic to whom you entrust your car will do his work and take responsibility for service and repairs. You count on him getting help if he can't do the job himself, and you expect him to have the necessary tools. And you don't want to hear any excuses about the garage's financial situation.

Unfortunately we sometimes come across staff in dementia care who think like this mechanic. They don't understand that it's their job to ensure that people with dementia have a good everyday life, good hygiene and a sense of being able to oversee their lives. And they have plenty of good excuses – for example that people with dementia are lacking in motivation, that there aren't enough resources, or that the necessary competence is lacking. This is obviously not OK.

We shall consider the tools and methods we need in order to fulfil the tasks we have as staff in everyday life. We have already looked at some of this in the first part of the book, but in the second part, we will get down to more practical details.

13

An Example from Everyday Life

RODDY

Roddy recently moved into a care home, after his beloved wife died, and he no longer could manage at home. Roddy has worked in the correctional system his whole life. He has been a conscientious man and held a position of leadership in the prison during the last years of his career. From the very first day, Roddy refuses to stay in his room; instead he goes into the office with the staff when they are going to have a meeting. A member of staff, Kate, takes him out to the others in the lounge and tells him to stay there. Roddy responds by telling her off, loudly. While the meeting is in progress, Roddy pilots three ladies into randomly chosen rooms and pushes a man in a wheelchair into the storeroom. When the staff come out of the office after the meeting, they hear someone calling for help from the storeroom. Roddy, meanwhile, is on his way down the other corridor pushing a lady in a wheelchair who is crying loudly: 'I don't want to come.' Roddy shouts at her: 'Be quiet and come along!'

Kate runs after him, takes hold of the wheelchair and says: 'You can't walk away with Doris.' Then Roddy gets upset and pushes Kate so that she falls over. He takes hold of the wheelchair again and carries on with Doris. Kate follows him, saying: 'Roddy, you have to stop! Doris doesn't want to go and you can't drive away with her. You can either sit and take it easy in the lounge or go to your room. But you can't push the others around. You're not the one in charge here!'

When she catches up with the wheelchair and driver she puts her hand on Roddy's shoulder. He then turns around and head-butts her. Kate's colleague Theresa presses the alarm button. Within a minute, three colleagues arrive, take hold of Roddy and push him to the floor. He spits, hisses and tries to bite them. The nurse calls the doctor and gets authorisation to give him a calming injection. After a while they put him in his bed. After the event, a meeting is held with the doctor and Roddy is put on anti-psychotic medication.

A CONFLICT

It's not so hard to understand this situation based on the principles we have considered so far. Kate works under the assumption that Roddy knows that he is not one of the staff. She therefore expects it to be sufficient if she takes him out of the office, into the lounge, and tells him to stay there. But her demand doesn't work quite as expected because Roddy doesn't sit down and relax. Obviously she hasn't presented her demand in a way that works.

When the staff meeting is over and the staff discover what Roddy is busy doing, Kate becomes authoritarian. By saying 'You can't!' and 'You're not the one in charge here!' she is setting boundaries. This is something that Roddy is not prepared for. In his world he is the boss, and he's in the process of creating order. When Kate's boundary-setting doesn't work, she reinforces it. She hasn't understood that Roddy only behaves well if he is able to do so. So actually

Kate's affect curve is on its way up before Roddy's curve is. When she sets the first boundary this functions as an affect trigger for Roddy. He doesn't understand what's going on, his frustration increases and he goes into the escalation phase. And Kate further increases his affect by going after him again and taking hold of him. This is too much for Roddy. He loses control.

In the situation that follows, the entire group of staff forget that Roddy is unable to cooperate as long as he doesn't have self-control. They deprive him of the possibility to cooperate, first by physically restraining him, and then by completely removing his self-control with a sedative injection. The only reason that Roddy has acted in the way he has is that he has tried to resolve the situation using the resources available to him.

Kate doesn't win. Nor does Roddy. Kate tries to win at first, but when Roddy pushes her, she probably realises that she hasn't. So she continues the conflict. And gets head-butted. Finally, after using violence, she and the rest of the staff feel that they eventually won. But that can be discussed. Roddy has clearly lost. But in fact so have the staff. They have missed the chance to get good cooperation with Roddy and his quality of life will be significantly affected for the worse, in the long run. Because of the anti-psychotic medication he is given, the risk is also high that he will die earlier than he otherwise would have. So who loses? Actually, everyone.

In this example the staff do not accomplish their task in a satisfactory manner. In other words, they have not fulfilled their contract with society. The result is that Roddy has a terrible experience and a worsened prognosis for the future. Who, then, is responsible for this? Unfortunately, we have to say the staff. And furthermore, there is nothing to suggest that anyone has learnt anything from the situation.

Situations like this arise all the time, in all care homes. We misunderstand. We expect too much of the abilities of the people with dementia who are in our care. We act impulsively instead of thinking things through. What is important then is that we become aware of the situation and make sure that it can't happen again. A problem that arises here, however, is that because of the power balance between the residents and us, we are the ones who will summarise what happened. Our version will be given the greatest weight.

In the example with Roddy and Kate, like most of us Kate will have difficulty in admitting that she had a part in escalating the situation with Roddy. She will have a tendency to defend her actions. Because she, just like Roddy, has actually only made use of solutions. The trouble is that she has much greater responsibility than Roddy in this situation, and so she should have found solutions that didn't create problems for him.

If we are to have a chance to improve, then there needs to be a context where situations like these can be discussed without placing shame on anyone in the staff.

In the short-term perspective, every time there has been a conflict between a staff-member and a person with dementia that has resulted in the person with dementia swearing, hitting staff, running away or throwing things around, it's a good idea for us to sit down and review the situation in the light of the affect-regulation model.

The questions we should ask ourselves in the different phases of the model are based on person-centred care and low-arousal thinking (key words are italicised). We will use the situation with Roddy as an example and go through the different phases in the affect regulation model step-by-step.

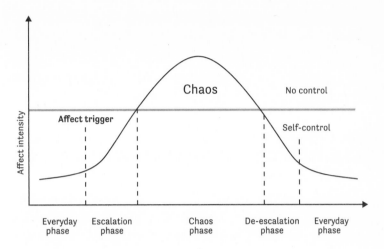

Figure 13.1 The affect regulation model

In the everyday calm phase, the staff ask themselves the following questions:

- Who said what?

- What did we expect Roddy to be able to do?

- Was Roddy able to do this?

- Were there adequate *structures* and *support* available to help Roddy to do what we expected him to?

- Was the environment *calm* enough?

- Did Roddy feel *included* in the context of which he was a part, or did he feel excluded?

- Did we do all we could to give Roddy a feeling of *belonging*?

- Did Roddy participate in what were for him *meaningful activities*?

Then the following questions are asked:

- Was it our behaviour that triggered Roddy's affect?

- If so, how can we make sure it doesn't happen again?

- Was there *warmth* and friendliness in our way of dealing with Roddy?

- How have we made sure that Roddy's level of *well-being* is high?

- Overall, are his basic psychological needs fulfilled?

- Should the *structures* and the *support* around Roddy be changed?

In the escalation phase, during which most of the conflict between Roddy and Kate takes place, the following questions are asked:

- What solutions did Roddy use?

- Would his *strategies for handling the situation* have been OK in his earlier life?

- Did he get the chance to *collect himself* and *maintain control*?

- Did we use strategies that focused on meeting Roddy in his own perception of the situation (*validation*)? Which?

- Was Roddy *treated* as an *equal cooperation partner*?

- Did we use solutions that caused problems for Roddy, which he then had to find solutions for? Which?

- Did we increase our *demands* in the escalation phase? How?

- Did we use any strategies to help Roddy *maintain self-control* in the escalation phase (such as creating distance, avoiding eye contact, turning aside)? Which?

- Did we use *body language* and a *tone of voice* that rather diminished Roddy's ability to maintain control (pronounced and insistent body language, direct, demanding eye contact, did we go closer to him, did we raise our voices, did we take hold of him)? Which?

- Did we use *distraction strategies* to actively help Roddy maintain his self-control? Which? What effect did they have?

In the chaos phase, the following questions are asked:

- Were we able to keep quiet while Roddy was in chaos?

- Was the situation dangerous?

- If it was a dangerous situation, was it interrupted in a quick, effective manner without increasing the level of conflict? How?

- Was it interrupted in such a way that Roddy's *well-being* was increased?

- Did our way of resolving the situation entail any *danger* for Roddy?

- If the situation was not dangerous, did we refrain from intervening?

- Did we use strategies to avoid increasing the chaos (no eye contact, distance, etc.)? Which?

In the de-escalation phase, the following questions are asked:

- Was Roddy given the space and quiet he needed to *land* in a good way?

- Did we do anything that caused the situation to escalate again (such as setting boundaries, reprimanding, instructing and pointing out negative consequences of the behaviour or making new demands before Roddy was ready)? What?

- Was *comfort* available?

- Did we succeed in supporting Roddy in his perception of the situation (*validation*)?

Finally we're back in the everyday calm phase, where the following questions are asked:

- Which *structures* must be changed in order for this not to happen again?

  ▸ Physical structures?

  ▸ Rule structures?

  ▸ Time-related structures?

- Do we have an *action plan* that we think will work if the same situation arises again?

These are not very difficult questions when it comes to the conflict between Roddy and Kate. When we go through them one by one, there isn't much that Kate did right. But since the objective of the questions is to work out how the staff as a whole can avoid a similar situation occurring in the future, the team's conversation shouldn't be about what Kate specifically did wrong. Rather, it should be about what they all can do next time a similar situation arises. This is called a *professionalisation process*, where the focus is moved from the individual to the method. It's actually not all that interesting to know why Kate did what she did, whether it was wrong, and what the consequences were. What is more interesting for Kate and her colleagues to know is what they can do next time it happens – so that they get better at their work. This means that in their discussions they shouldn't discuss who is to blame, but only the method. Their conversation should preferably lead to a change in their way of working. But also to an action plan that everyone follows next time they find themselves in something that could turn into a conflict situation like the one they have discussed.

The changes in routine that Kate and her colleagues need to make after the situation with Roddy are quite straightforward. They formulate the following points:

- Roddy must never be left alone with the other older people, there must always be a member of staff nearby who can maintain the daily structure and care work – even if there is a staff meeting.

- Before staff meetings we will make sure that Roddy is busy with a good and meaningful activity.

- If he tries to follow us in to the staff meeting, we have two possibilities:

  ▸ We assign a member of staff to help him back to his activity. Only when he is back in his place can the member of staff return to the meeting.

  ▸ Roddy is present at the meeting.

- We will meet Roddy in his perception of reality during the entire course of events.

- We will not raise our voices.

- We will not take hold of Roddy.

When we have been through a difficult situation, it is always relevant to talk about what we as staff should do, and it is important for that conversation to be received in a good way by everyone on the team. This doesn't mean that we must have a talk with the relevant member of staff about what he did (that would be based on the belief that the person will learn from the situation and could have acted differently, which is not relevant). What is important is that we develop good methods and routines for creating calm in situations where there previously has been unrest. For example, it might be a good idea to create an opportunity for the older person to withdraw and be alone if he wants to, or to offer to do a quiet activity together with him that we know he enjoys.

One small thing. Sometimes in our work we hear the argument that you're supposed to feel bad when things have gone wrong, because this reduces the risk that it will happen again. We totally disagree. We needn't worry that the risk of violence will increase just because we got the person to feel secure and content after the conflict. To think that a person should experience negative consequences after negative behaviour builds on the idea that the person learns from the experience. This we have been through already. Dementia means that you no longer learn. Besides, there are far too many negative experiences associated with the violence itself for the whole to be seen as a positive situation. People with dementia don't really want to fight, they want to behave. If they fight, it's because that's what gives most meaning in the situation they are in. And if that's the case, then maybe it's better to change what gives meaning to the person before the next time it happens. This we can do with an action plan.

ACTION PLANS

Action plans for conflict situations are simple lists of how we as staff should act when a conflict is developing. They should be personal, in other words be concerned with a single individual. Many no doubt think that action plans are just one more form of unnecessary documentation. It is then important to remember that we don't make action plans for situations that have not occurred, and that many of the people we care for don't need an action plan, because we don't have any conflicts with them that we can't handle without one.

The process of making an action plan starts with making a list of warning behaviours, in other words behaviours that the person displays when things are about to go wrong. It may be that he talks a lot, walks about, raises his voice, or chews his fingers. These are behaviours that the person doesn't usually exhibit but that have been noticed on other occasions just before things went wrong.

A good action plan has five steps:

1. *Make room to validate the person's own strategies for handling the situation.* If that doesn't help, move on to step 2.

2. *Use simple distractions that have worked before.* This could mean going over to the person and just be nearby in order to create calm with one's own calmness. To gently and in a relaxed way help him move on with his day, or something similar. If this doesn't help or if the person reacts negatively to this, move on to step 3.

3. *Use active distractions that have worked before.* This could mean talking to the person about something they like, joking gently with them, or something like that. The focus is to create good contact. It could also mean offering something to eat or a cup of coffee, encouraging and acknowledging the person as a person, or initiating some form of cooperation. This should be done in a friendly and quiet tone and with focus on the person's self-control. If this doesn't work, move on to step 4.

4. *Use calming actions.* If the person is near or above the affect regulation line, that is to say in chaos, then the level of affect is so high that the person can seldom be reached with normal pedagogical strategies. Instead of then using a lot of words to try and reduce the affect – regardless of whether the intention is validation or different degrees of distraction – it is more effective to act calmly, maintain a physical distance and avoid eye contact. It is important to have a relaxed body language directed away from the person in affect, for example by sitting on the floor or sofa. This signals that one is calm and, not least, that one has time. One can also dispel the affect by physically leaving the room for a while, in order to try again a bit later or to let another member of staff try. If this is not enough, move on to step 5.

5. *Interrupt the situation or wait until it ends on its own.* A good rule of thumb is that people only have the strength to throw furniture around for a couple of minutes. In such a situation, handling the conflict usually consists of making sure there are no other residents nearby (offer them another activity). One can

also let a little time go by without any further actions, in order to give the affect time to subside to the point where the person is open to renewed efforts. In some cases, for example when the behaviour is dangerous, such as during a violent fight between two people with dementia, it may be good to physically separate the combatants with the aid of movement (not holding, which increases the conflict and the chaos) and quickly letting go again. This can be repeated several times at short intervals if necessary, until the person who is in chaos begins to de-escalate. Intervening with movement is a method that was developed by British psychologist Andy McDonnell. It builds on the principle of moving with a person's movements and guiding them by reinforcing the movements when they are going in the same direction as the person is moving, letting go after a couple of seconds. One should not use force, in other words, as it only increases the level of conflict and brings with it the risk that the person will lose his balance, with the real risk of broken arms and the like. And no-one wants to see that happen. The method of following along with a movement is tremendously distracting, but must naturally still be considered as use of physical force. It must therefore not become an everyday method, only a method to use in emergencies.

The reason we have selected just five steps builds on the experience of the staff at the Disability Centre, Malmö, Sweden. After some experimentation, they found that when using five steps, followed as described above, they very seldom reached step five. Using more steps or fewer steps more often led to chaos behaviour.

It is useful to have a list of distractions that have worked before. It often happens that different members of staff use different distractions. It can therefore be helpful to collect all the distractions that work on a single list. In this way, one can get very useful action plans.

ACTION PLAN FOR RODDY

If we go back to Roddy, the staff's action plan for him could look something like this:

1. *Stay calm*. If Roddy starts to get annoyed it is usually because he hasn't understood. Talk to him based on his perception of the situation (for example that he is a manager in the correctional system, or that he wants to help). Make sure that the one he is wheeling away has a good experience and doesn't become anxious. Here are some concrete phrases one could use:

   ▶ 'Hello Roddy, my name is XXXX.' (A hand is stretched out to encourage Roddy to put out his hand.)

   ▶ 'Hello Roddy, here you are. Where are you heading?'

   ▶ 'May I talk to Doris for a bit before you carry on?'

   If Roddy gets more riled up, move on to step 2.

2. *Walk along with Roddy*. Speak calmly both to him and the person he is driving away. Help him stop and go back by speaking from the perspective of how he is perceiving the situation. For example: 'Good thing you came Roddy, I have something I would very much like you to help me with; would you mind coming with me to the lounge?' Or, more briefly: 'Good thing you came,

I need your help. Come, quickly.' If this doesn't work, or if he reacts negatively to this, move on to step 3.

3. *Talk to Roddy about his car.* He had a Mercedes that he really liked and spent a lot of time on. This puts him in a good mood and makes him willing to cooperate. Or discuss the local football club. Roddy has always been a football supporter and always reacts positively to talk about football. By talking to him about cars or football, it is usually possible to get him to turn back. Another good method is to say that it's time for a break and that coffee is being served in the lounge, and pour him a cup of coffee. That nearly always works. Keep a friendly tone. Another method is to use an object, such as a towel or a box, and ask: 'Could you please hold this, Roddy?' If that doesn't help, move on to step 4.

4. *Let Roddy keep going*, and start distraction manoeuvres again when he is on his way back to the lounge to fetch a new person. It is easier to distract him when he isn't wheeling someone away. Preferably the member of staff who talks to him on his way back should be a different person to the one who first tried. Also, make sure that the one he has driven away is properly taken care of and helped back to the lounge after a while. If Roddy is too wound up or is already in chaos, move on to step 5.

5. *Begin by moving* the other residents out of the lounge and into their own rooms. If there is no-one left for Roddy to wheel away or follow out, then he usually settles down. After a little while, a new person from the staff can offer him an activity that he likes. Wait another ten minutes after this, then bring back those residents who would like to be there to the lounge.

14

People With Great Social Needs

DENNIS

Dennis is a youngish man of 45 who stays in respite care one week every month. The staff have a hard time activating him and they are under the impression that he provokes them deliberately. They say that when they go for walks with Dennis next to open fields, he runs away from them just to annoy them. He also often kicks at things he comes across while walking in the nearby residential neighbourhood.

When Dennis is in the home and comes out into the corridor, he takes running jumps to hit the lamps hanging from the ceiling. When he is sitting in the lounge, he puts a leg out when someone goes past. As if that was not enough, he also creeps up behind the female staff and when he gets the chance, grabs their bra bands from behind, stretches them, and laughs loudly when he lets go.

Dennis is a social person who loves social intercourse. He just isn't very good at it any more. So he does what he can to connect with the staff. Working with Dennis is a bit different to working with most other people with dementia, partly because of his age. He has considerably more energy than most people in their eighties.

The staff think that Dennis is teasing. This is a very interesting word. Because it's possible to tease in the sense of bullying, and to tease in the sense of flirting. From a moral perspective, we look very differently at these two types of teasing. It's OK to tease as part of flirting if kept at a level where both parties think it's fun. But bullying is never OK. Dennis isn't able to keep his teasing at an acceptable level because he can't read nuances in the way required to tease in a joking manner. One has to be able to adjust one's teasing depending on how the other person takes it. This is why the staff think that he is teasing in a way that is reminiscent of bullying. Naturally this is a problem, because they are ascribing him a negative intention. That he wants to annoy the staff.

In reality, Dennis wants to have a good contact with them. He wants to get a feel for them. Some people are introverted and prefer to be by themselves, while others are extroverted and need contact with other people in order to feel that they exist. Many of us need both, partly being in contact with other people, but also sometimes being allowed to be alone. A few prefer to be alone all the time, and a few others have such great social needs that they can't stand to be alone at all. We can see it as having different levels of need for other people. Presumably Dennis belongs to the group that has great social needs and so he cannot be alone.

The problem is that with the progress of his dementia he has lost his social skills. He is now a man with great social needs and very little social competence. This is a bad combination and there are not many people with dementia who have it. But those who do take enormous space, and are unfortunately more often the object of scolding and reprimands than others. Yet another factor involved is that they are difficult to be with. We have a tendency to try to avoid them and perhaps turn our backs to them to some extent. But unfortunately, great social needs in a person with dementia and staff who turn their backs are a really bad combination.

MARJORIE

Marjorie is seen by the staff as extremely demanding of attention. She sits in her wheelchair in the lounge, the whole time half-crying: 'Hello, hello, come and help me.' Zadie goes over to Marjorie and asks what she can do to help. Marjorie answers, puzzled: 'Nothing. Do I need help?' Zadie says: 'Marjorie, you're always crying for help. You must understand that this disturbs the others, and that you must be quiet when you don't need help.' 'OK, I certainly will,' answers Marjorie.

Zadie goes away and soon Marjorie begins again: 'Hello, hello, come and help me.' Zadie turns abruptly and says to Marjorie: 'That's enough. Didn't you hear what I said? If you don't stop that, we'll take you off to your room!'

Marjorie has the same great social needs that Dennis has. She finds it difficult to be alone. So she tries to make contact. For her, just as for Dennis, it doesn't matter if the contact is of poor quality, as long as it's there.

There are some professionals who say that a behaviour will end if you just ignore it. We don't think this is a good method. To be ignored is not to be seen, validated, met with respect and acceptance, supported or included, and all the other key words that are so central in person-centred care. Neither is it effective. Often a behaviour will increase in a person if we ignore them. The social needs don't diminish just because they are not acknowledged. Therefore, neither Dennis nor Marjorie should be ignored. And the staff who work with them should not work with their backs turned. Both Dennis and Marjorie need staff who prioritise contact with them.

Below, we describe some ways of getting people who have great social needs to function well:

- *Fill the need.* This is best accomplished by the staff dedicating time to the person several times a day. During that time, the focus should be on good emotional contact, for example with humour or interesting topics of discussion, or with someone like Dennis whose language skills are no longer very good, running races or the like. A half-hour a few times a day is time well spent. Altogether, it takes considerably less time when it is the staff who take the social initiatives.

- *Take social initiatives before the person does.* Both Dennis' and Marjorie's social initiatives are of rather poor quality. Therefore the staff should remember to pre-empt them, since they have considerably better social competence, which means that they can take much better social initiatives than Dennis or Marjorie can. That's why they can't work with their backs turned.

- *Improve the quality of the interaction.* In the situations above, it is Dennis and Marjorie who act first. The situations consist of their initiatives and the staff's reactions. Their initiative and the staff's reaction. And so it goes on. If instead the staff had been able to get a grip on the situation and improve its quality, they would have met Dennis and Marjorie's needs a little better. For example, by continuing to converse with them instead of just answering. When Marjorie says 'Do I need help?' they could very well start joking with her about what she might need help with. Then they would have improved the quality of the interaction and had a good and productive conversation. This would have increased both Marjorie's and the staff's sense of well-being.

- *Take control.* If it feels difficult to always talk about the same thing, one has to try to find a new subject to talk about. That's why it's a good idea to have a few topics or activities prepared in advance for use when needed. Or one can make use of strong distractions, using concrete objects, for example, or do something surprising like singing a song.

- For some people it is effective if, instead of talking, one *transfers the need for social contact over to a clearly physical and social contact*, so-called deep pressure (for example pressing down on the shoulders) or massage. This way they feel themselves through the physical contact.

- *Decide who among the staff will be the one to focus on the person.* One of the mechanisms that arises when you work with your back turned is that you often delay in answering or reacting. You simply hope that a colleague will deal with the situation. So you not only turn your back, you also do so a little longer than you otherwise would. This means that the time it takes to handle a difficult situation is often a bit longer than usual. By ensuring that in every shift there is someone with primary responsible for the person, you can interact with them in a better way. This also means that the other staff get more peace and quiet to perform their duties.

- *Take the person with you to a place or situation where the behaviour doesn't disturb others or fits in better.*

Let it take the time it takes. If you try to minimise the time it takes to work with a person with great social needs, it will most often take more time.

15

Inappropriate Behaviour

IRVING AND CHARLOTTE

Beth has died, and on a frosty February morning she is picked up by the undertaker. The residents and staff gather in the lounge to sing a psalm. Staff from other departments have also come to say goodbye to Beth. One of the residents, Irving, looks with interest at the female employees who have just arrived. When Beth is brought in and it's time to sing, Irving says in a loud, clear voice: 'I want pussy, I want pussy now.' The staff members who are standing with Irving say: 'We're just going to sing first.'

Another resident, Charlotte, goes over to one of the women among the staff, lifts up her blouse and looks underneath while saying: 'What bra are you wearing?' Then she pulls her own blouse over her head to show her own bra and says: 'Mine has lace and I'm wearing a thong.' After a bit of a tumult the singing for Beth is over and, while everyone is standing by the hearse to say a final goodbye, Irving says loudly: 'Shit! I think someone has died.'

This is a fantastic situation. And a good example of how as staff we dearly like to maintain traditions and normal ways of doing things, without always thinking through what this entails in the form of demands on and expectations of people with dementia. This whole situation places some general demands on the residents:

- They must understand that someone has died.

- They must have a general idea of normal behaviour when someone has died so that they can participate without disturbing.

- They must remember what they are doing until it is all over.

- They must have good enough social skills to adjust their behaviour:

  ▸ If someone has died they should act in a dignified manner.

  ▸ In a situation where there are several people around they should not talk about wanting pussy or pull up their blouse. These actions belong in other settings.

  ▸ They should understand their own social position in relation to the others present.

As the situation around Beth's farewell develops it becomes clear that the demands are too high, at least for Irving and Charlotte. They do what is meaningful to them in the situation. In such a setting, the staff can't keep on singing and pretend that nothing is going on. They are at work. Of course they can't expect that Irving and Charlotte will suddenly be able to behave themselves.

In this case the staff do a good job. They take things as they come. Maybe things aren't as ceremonious as they might have been. But everyone participates. That is valuable in itself, both for those who are present and for the future. If the staff had started by sending Irving and Charlotte off to their rooms when they were going to sing for Beth, then there would have been a risk that they would start excluding Irving and Charlotte from more and more activities. Maybe they would have started to think that they were disturbing them in their work. But that would have been to rob both Irving and Charlotte of a portion of their personalities.

The goal in care for older people is for them all to be able to participate on equal terms, for as long as they are able and gain something from it. We just need to take responsibility the whole way through, so that things turn out well and lead to good quality of life.

16

Relatives Are People Too

DALE

Dale, who is a relative, arrives unannounced on a visit to the day centre where his uncle John has just started. Dale speaks very quickly and says: 'I just want to see if anything happens, because if he's just going to sit and stare he might as well stay at home.'

Emily, who works at the day centre, explains that they have just arrived and are about to have breakfast. Dale gets agitated and speaks more loudly: 'I give him breakfast at 6 o'clock and then the domiciliary care helper comes at 8 and gives him breakfast again, and now he's going to have it one more time, he'll get much too fat and in the end he won't be able to walk any more.' He carries on: 'Yes, I've complained about the domiciliary care. They buy all kinds of food that he can't eat, it's the kind of stuff they eat and drink themselves. And by the way, John isn't very demented, because he remembers names.'

Emily invites him to sit and chat for a while. She begins the conversation by saying: 'Are you angry with the domiciliary care?'

'Yes, I'm not allowed to be his guardian, and you know what, I had a stroke a few years ago and then John took care of me and thanks to him I am able to walk again today, and I promised that I would take care of him if he needed it, but the domiciliary care won't let me.'

He pulls a roll of mints from his pocket and says: 'This is for you, you're the nicest person I've met.' He looks around. 'When the weather gets better he can come outside and sit out here, I know he'd like that, I'm off now, thanks for the chat.'

ANNE

Anne's mother Bridget has just moved into a care home. Anne comes for a visit. She meets Susan who works there and asks how things are going. Susan is not quite sure how to answer, since she has heard that Anne is a nurse and that she has asked the evening shift some critical questions. Susan answers: 'I think it's going very well; Bridget is happy, after all.'

Anne replies a little suspiciously: 'What do you mean happy? My mother can't possibly be happy, she's cried every time I've visited her.' She goes on to ask: 'How did she sleep last night?'

Susan hasn't read whether or not Bridget slept well last night, but she hasn't heard anything about her lying awake, so she says: 'I haven't heard anything.'

Anne says: 'If you haven't heard anything, then how can you take care of my mother? It is actually important for people with dementia to get a good sleep, otherwise their behaviour can be misinterpreted. Do you know how much she's eaten, then?'

Now Susan is feeling cornered and forced to defend herself, so she says: 'Well, during my shifts she has been at the table at every meal, but I don't know how much she has eaten, but neither is she exactly skinny so she will probably be OK. I don't know how it is during the other shifts, it often happens that someone on the evening shift forgets to write something.'

Anne says in a very decided tone of voice: 'My mother needs someone to sit with her in the late afternoon, otherwise she gets totally confused and starts to cry. I'm counting on you being able to do this. Now I'll go down and see how she is.'

The stories about Dale and Anne include many of the themes that we come across when we are out doing training.

Relatives have witnessed their near and dear ones fall apart, till they no longer resemble the people they once knew. It can be equated to the person dying. But that has not happened, so the relatives are in mourning, but can't mourn.

The relatives often have a bad conscience. Maybe because they promised to take care of the person, but maybe also because they think they could have done more while the person still lived at home. Not shouted so much, been a bit more tolerant. Maybe they also feel bad because they can't take being there for very long. Many relatives can't stand visiting for very long, and as soon as they leave they get a bad conscience.

The relatives often have an underlying anxiety that is due to them having handed over their loved one to the goodwill of the public sector. You wonder whether the staff are doing a good enough job, whether your relatives will be hurt or sad, whether they will run away, or whether they get enough to eat and drink. This is a constant worry that no-one can completely eliminate, but it can be alleviated.

As staff, we must listen for this kind of sorrow, guilty conscience and anxiety. If the relative is not accommodated in this, for example if the staff answer as in the case described above, then the relative feels powerless. She feels that she has not been listened to in her anxiety, sorrow and guilty conscience, and in her powerlessness begins to point out faults and shortcomings, and to use authoritativeness (such as nurses' training in the example), and it will no doubt all end in one or more complaints. And most likely Bridget will not get any better nursing and care, let alone any good visits with her daughter, where they can just be mother and daughter.

The staff feel scrutinised, and as if people think they can't do their job well enough. They feel powerless about not being able to please the relative, no matter what they do. They will try to avoid the relative, place the blame on each other (in Susan's case on the evening shift) or start talking about inadequate resources. Within the staff group, private stories may start going around about how the relative doesn't understand her mother, how she is always sad when the daughter is there, or how the relative is too demanding and wants special treatment that negatively affects the others. Maybe a basic story about how the relative's visits are bad for the person in care and how the staff are much better at being with her. These stories have to do with seeing the relatives not as people, but as relatives. In person-centred care, relatives are also people and deserve to be treated as people, not as representing the role of a relative.

As staff we have to be professional and understand what is at stake for the relatives. We also need to provide guidance on how a relative can have the best possible visit. Because having relatives for a visit can never be replaced by nursing staff and has great importance for the patient's quality of life.

We should naturally also be able to give relevant answers to the questions posed by the relatives. Susan ends up in a situation where she feels cornered and forced to defend herself. This happens because she doesn't succeed in getting Anne to trust her and relinquish her authority. Anne doesn't feel that Susan is worthy of trust. In this situation Susan can react in different ways:

- She can become confrontational and refer Anne to the management with any complaints. Behind this lies the idea that Susan as a member of staff should not have to be the object of a relative's anger. The result will probably be that Anne's level of confidence in the competence of the staff will drop even lower. So not a good idea.

- She can become even more fearful of conflict and more evasive next time she meets Anne. This will also reduce Anne's confidence in the ability of the staff to create a good life for Bridget. Not a good idea either.

- She can choose to be clear and professional. This means giving clear answers to Anne's questions if she knows the answers, and promising to find out right away if she doesn't.

The last method is without doubt the one to be preferred. Relatives need to meet staff who both treat them as real people and who give the impression that they know what they are doing, and are in control over what is happening to the older person.

To get off to a good start in cooperating with a relative:

- Begin by meeting with the relative. Give them the opportunity to tell their story and explain their wishes. When did the relative discover that there was something wrong with the older person? How did the relative tackle all the difficult situations that led up to them seeking help? What was it that forced them to give up? How are they mourning? What is their biggest concern right now? What do they hope for from their visit? How do they want you to work together?

- After that a different conversation should be held in which the staff learn about the older person's life history, for use in thinking forwards in nursing and care. We use the life history as a reference in creating a context for the older person. These two conversations should preferably take place on separate occasions.

- Suggest some activities that the relative can do together with their loved one. It is better to drink coffee together than to tidy the room when visiting, for example. Suggest activities that can take place even if the older person doesn't seek contact with their relative or doesn't want to have anything to do with them. And naturally we must use pedagogical guidance to support the relative who feels rejected, for example if their spouse has found someone else to walk with hand-in-hand in the home. This can be a very painful thing for the healthy partner and requires support from the staff.

- And naturally we must maintain an ongoing dialogue with the relative about our cooperation.

Summary

Relatives are people too and must be met with the same respect as the older people we are responsible for. This means that we must show an understanding of the relative's situation and sorrow, and create the necessary conditions for the relative to be able to trust us. This we do best through good care of the older person and clear communication with the relative.

17

Always Exclude the Possibility that It Could Be Somatic

SALLY

Sally's dementia has deteriorated quickly. A week ago she was going around participating in activities and was usually in a good mood, but now she just sits in a wheelchair wailing loudly: 'But help me, but help me then.'

The staff have been discussing whether sedative medication might help. She seems anxious. Her wailing is also very disturbing for the other residents. It spreads anxiety. In order to decide whether to start medication, the doctor asks the staff a number of questions. In the conversation it comes up that Sally is constipated. She receives an enema and later the same day she is the good old Sally again, who walks around and is in a good mood.

THE POWER OF SOMATICS

Most of the literature that exists about behaviour that challenges in dementia begins by describing behaviour that challenges that occurs because the person in question, above and beyond his dementia, doesn't feel well. Because the person feels sad, can't eat properly, or for other somatic reasons.

We have chosen to end this book by discussing this problem area since up to half of the behavioural problems that occur in people with dementia can be relieved by seeing to it that they have everything they need to feel well.

We have intentionally saved this for the end because the book is actually about managing behaviour that challenges. In other words we expect that you as a reader have eliminated somatic causes for the various types of behaviour and that you have chosen to read this book for other reasons. But to be on the safe side, we still want to have a look at what can be done to discover potential somatic problems that can cause behaviour that challenges in people with dementia.

We who work in older care are usually so used to the development of dementia that we tend to assume that it is the dementia that is the cause every time things go downhill for one of the older people. Possibly because people with incipient dementia can have difficulty in describing somatic symptoms. They may not even understand themselves why they don't feel well. Everyone behaves differently when they have physical symptoms. We are more easily irritated when we are in pain, we become apathetic when we have a fever, and we find it harder to concentrate when we desperately need to urinate. In people with dementia, there is a risk that physical symptoms such as these are first noticed through behavioural changes. Behavioural changes that we sometimes call behaviour that challenges.

Sally's story contains rule number 1 when it comes to somatics: if the condition of a person with dementia changes in just a few days or weeks, it is not due to the dementia but to something somatic.

It is important to keep your eyes open for the following somatic symptoms since they can cause changes in behaviour:

- Does the person have a bladder infection, pneumonia or other infection? These conditions can easily occur without a fever.

- Has the person had enough to drink? Since there are many different shifts over a 24-hour period, it is impossible to accurately say whether a person has had enough liquids unless a liquids chart is maintained. In case of uncertainty, the person's liquid intake should be recorded.

- Is the person constipated? Here the same thing applies. It is important to record when the person has had a bowel movement in order to be sure. A person can very well pass a thin, grainy stool but still be constipated. In really severe constipation, there may be constant leakage of a little runny stool, which, as it were, leaks out around the constipation.

- Does the person appear to be in pain? Most older people have daily pains that can noticeably worsen their condition and, in the worst cases, lead to delirium. People with dementia can seldom express their pain; instead they often react with anxiety, self-stimulating behaviour or aggressiveness.

- Is the person's blood sugar too high or too low?

- Is the person getting enough oxygen? If not, the cause could be poor circulation, low blood values or poor lung function.

- Does the person have any other deficiencies? If a deficiency is suspected, it is always good to do a proper medical check-up.

- Does the person have problems with their metabolism?

- Is the person's daily rhythm disrupted? A disturbed daily rhythm can have many causes, including pain, constipation, blood-sugar problems and thirst.

- Is the person suffering from poisoning? This includes interactions and side effects of medications. Many of the substances used for somatic conditions, such as diuretics, heart medications, Parkinson's medications and drugs for rheumatism, include confusion (disorientation) as a fairly common side effect. If a person is taking more than 3–5 medicines, then the risk of side effects and detrimental interactions increases.

Untreated, all these conditions can lead to the person being in danger of their life.

CONRAD

Conrad recently moved into the care home. He came directly from the hospital. He sits in a wheelchair, doesn't speak, and seems very apathetic. He sits in his wheelchair all day long, watching life go on around him. If there is nothing to look at, he sits slumped over. Conrad is receiving two kinds of anti-psychotic drugs, but since he doesn't seem to be psychotic, a reduction in dose is started. A week later the staff are having a breakfast meeting. In comes Conrad. He has walked from his room down to the office. 'There's a bit of poo here,' he says and points at his nappy. He would like some help with this. The reduction in medication has led to Conrad being able to walk around and say what he wants. The staff think it's magic.

CALMING MEDICINE

The story about Conrad contains rule number 2 with regard to somatics: psychotropic drugs have no effect on dementia symptoms, but instead they have a strong sedative effect on the brain and tend to accumulate in the body.

Psychotropic drugs, such as neuroleptics (anti-psychotic medication) or benzodiazepines (anxiety-relieving and calming medication), are often prescribed when a person is considered to have behaviour that challenges that can't be managed. Maybe because we think that the behaviour is not the result of the dementia, but rather of some psychiatric symptom, or of co-morbidities. In the field of medicine as a whole it is primarily in psychiatry that one encounters patients with behavioural symptoms, and they are most often treated with neuroleptics and benzodiazepines.

When we who work in care of older people contact a doctor because we have an older person with behaviour that challenges, we are already thinking that the problem is likely to be psychiatric in nature. And the doctor does what he has learnt during his training: he prescribes medicine. But when we see behavioural changes in a person with dementia, if we examine the symptoms from the perspective of what we know about different dementia illnesses, then there is seldom anything to indicate that we are dealing with anxiety or a psychotic condition.

High-quality person-centred care depends on people with dementia not being treated with neuroleptics and benzodiazepines that they don't need, because the medicines cause additional impairment in function by numbing the brain (which already has difficulty functioning). There is also research to show that the medication itself carries an increased risk of early death. So instead of medicating for behaviour that challenges, action plans should be developed so that such behaviour can be managed and prevented. And when we succeed in this, it can feel like pure magic.

There are plenty of stories similar to the ones of Sally and Conrad, in which a person's behaviour has changed markedly, and where discovery and management of a somatic cause has resolved the situation.

The somatic aspects are of course also important to consider in relation to our daily work with the affect regulation model that we looked at earlier in the book. Somatic causes (e.g. that a person didn't sleep well the night before, infection, pain or hunger) can contribute to loss of control or can result in the threshold at which this happens being considerably lower than normal.

We can see somatic symptoms as a kind of stress. And if we want to be successful in working with a person who is stressed, it is often a good idea to begin by reducing the person's stress levels. Somatic symptoms, such as sleep problems, pain, constipation and hunger, are strong stress factors. They are also what we call basic stress factors. That means that they affect the person's level of functioning the whole time. For example, a person who has slept poorly will have a harder time in managing the coming day.

This means that we should always identify somatic problems first and treat them before starting on more pedagogical methods. A good approach and well-considered pedagogy just don't work as well when a person has somatic symptoms. We have repeatedly been called in as consultants to cases where staff felt forced to use physical force and restraint in order to manage personal hygiene for people with dementia. With appropriate pain relief, this has suddenly been possible to do without any problem, using only encouragement and a friendly attitude. In the words of Danish geriatric psychiatrist Nils Christian Gulmann: 'Everything is somatic until proved otherwise.'

Summary

In many cases, behaviour that challenges is due to a somatic problem. To identify whether this is the case we need to know two rules: 1) if there have been changes in the person's condition during the past few days or weeks, it is not due to the dementia but due to something somatic; 2) psychotropic drugs have no effect on dementia symptoms; instead they have a strong sedative effect on the brain and tend to accumulate in the body, resulting in increased side effects.

Part 3

Extra Material

Types of Dementia

ALZHEIMER DEMENTIA

Alzheimer dementia, or Alzheimer's disease, is the most common type of dementia. More than half of all patients with dementia have Alzheimer dementia. The pattern begins with atrophy (reduced brain tissue) in the part of the brain that deals with spatial relationships, memory and learning. Later the atrophy spreads to most of the brain.

The first symptoms of a person with Alzheimer dementia are often that he can no longer find his way and that he misplaces things, for example putting his slippers in the fridge. After a while, the symptoms follow one after the other:

- Spatial perception is often seriously affected. This means that the staff have to help the person find his way around, and to find the way back to his room.

- The person has difficulty in finding the right words, at first especially nouns. For example, the person might say 'the thing you stir with' when he means a teaspoon. Language difficulties become more and more severe the further the disease progresses, and eventually the person will have great difficulty in expressing himself and in understanding what other people are saying.

- The person has difficulty in understanding more complex sensory impressions. This can mean, that they don't know what things are for. For example, a vase on the floor can be taken for a toilet bowl and so the person urinates in it.

- The person is affected by apraxia. This involves difficulty in performing complex actions such as getting dressed.

- The person has difficulty in recognising faces, sometimes even his own reflection in the mirror. Therefore a person with Alzheimer dementia may sometimes have long conversations with his reflection in a mirror, or in a window after nightfall.

The personality of people with Alzheimer dementia is relatively intact well into the course of the disease and so they often react in the same way that they have done in the past. Most of them can also maintain good relationships well into the course of the disease. It is not unusual for them to have good social competence and the ability to read emotions and moods well into the development of dementia. This is especially relevant when working according to the low-arousal approach, in which one seeks to influence moods and affects in the people with dementia that one is working with.

An important task for all who work with this group is to create security and comfort for them when the world is collapsing around them and they no longer can remember who or where they are. This often creates anxiety. Anxiety in combination with the weakened memory and the lost capacity for learning means that people with Alzheimer dementia need the same comforting talk over and over again. This is something the staff must take into account. It is common for people with this type of dementia to get angry if they feel unsuccessful when we place too high demands on them or want to make decisions for them. So it's a good idea to work in such a way that we create a sense of security and a good atmosphere.

VASCULAR DEMENTIA

Vascular dementia is the second most common type of dementia. Between 20 and 25 per cent of all people with dementia have this type. Vascular dementia actually consists of lots of small brain injuries caused by either oxygen deficiency or small haemorrhages in the brain. This means that the damage can appear in many different areas of the brain and so lead to different symptoms. Common symptoms include:

- Language disturbances.

- Perceptual disturbances.

- Reduced physical strength. The person becomes weak and may have difficulty walking, and may wet themselves.

- Memory difficulties in which the person has trouble remembering something he has just experienced or learnt. However, there is no difficulty remembering old knowledge.

- Slower processing ability.

- Difficulties in concentrating.

- Reduced initiative.

- Failing judgment and oversight.

- Difficulty in regulating one's affect, which means that various emotional expressions are frequent, such as tears. Depression is also quite common.

FRONTOTEMPORAL DEMENTIA

Between 3 and 5 per cent of all people with dementia have frontotemporal dementia. Some of them are affected particularly by disturbances in behaviour and personality, while others have most difficulty with language and memory.

The first group quickly loses interest in things that they were previously absorbed by, and lose their relationships. They often have difficulties in empathising with other people's experiences and are therefore seen as indifferent to others, even to their own relatives. This is probably the thing that is most difficult for both staff and relatives to deal with. In other types of dementia the person often continues to be the same person, but in frontotemporal dementia many have such marked changes in personality that they seem to be different people. Therefore one must act quite differently towards a person with frontotemporal dementia than towards someone with Alzheimer dementia. A person with frontotemporal dementia can't read the staff member's mood and adjust his behaviour accordingly. This means that one needs to speak in very concrete terms, and say what the person should do and what is going to happen.

Besides these symptoms, the following are also common in frontotemporal dementia:

- Difficulty in concentrating.

- Difficulty in oversight and planning.

- Impulsive behaviour. For example the person might say loudly: 'What a fat pig' when he sees a fat person.

- Things tend to develop a summoning nature for them. For example, the person can't keep from sitting down on a chair when he sees one, opening and closing doors, or running around in the corridors.

- Development of compulsive behaviour. This may be expressed as excessive washing, having a problem going through doors, or checking repeatedly that the exterior door is closed.

- Personality changes. The person often has a hard time seeing things from other people's perspective and their behaviour may therefore seem egotistic and inappropriate.

People with frontotemporal dementia can become angry if one says 'no' to them or sets boundaries. Therefore it is important to stay calm and use distractions.

In people with frontotemporal dementia who get severe difficulties with language and memory, speech becomes hesitant, choppy and full of repetition; in the end they often stop talking altogether.

LEWY BODY DEMENTIA

Lewy Body dementia is as common as frontotemporal dementia. The disease begins with attention difficulties, and during the course of the illness the person can start to be absent for hours at a time. In the final stages, the person can have periods where the degree of consciousness is so low that the staff think he has died, and raise the alarm. Other common symptoms are:

- Very realistic visual hallucinations. The person often sees people and animals, but without being bothered by them emotionally in the way that people with psychoses are. It can be distressing for the person, but not so anxiety-ridden and paranoia-oriented as in the case of psychosis. Because of the hallucinations, some are unfortunately given inappropriate antipsychotic medication, which has no positive effect and is actually life-threatening for them.

- Motor skill disturbances which, among other things, often make the person stiff.

- Difficulties with spatial understanding similar to what one sees in Alzheimer dementia.

People with Lewy Body dementia don't have as much trouble with their memory as people with other types of dementia, but they may have difficulty in learning new things.

OTHER TYPES OF DEMENTIA

There are many other types of dementia, but they are less common than those described above. Some are substance-related, such as alcohol dementia or painter's syndrome (chronic solvent-induced encephalopathy). Others are illnesses that affect the whole nervous system, such as Parkinson's disease, Huntington's disease and multiple sclerosis. In addition, there are certain expressions of dementia that are connected with Down's syndrome and other so-called developmental disabilities.

As stated, the purpose of this book is not to provide detailed information about dementia illnesses, but about how we who work in older care can think and act. When we are given an assignment involving a person with dementia, however, it is always a good idea to first make oneself familiar with the type of dementia that the person has. More detailed information is available on the internet, for example at the National Institute of Neurological Disorders and Stroke website or in books such as Husain and Schott (2016).

REFERENCES

Husain, M. and Schott, J.M. (eds) (2016) *Oxford Textbook of Cognitive Neurology and Dementia.* Oxford: Oxford University Press.

National Institute of Neurological Disorders and Stroke (2016) www.ninds.nih.gov.

Person-centred Care

The idea behind person-centred care is that the person comes before the diagnosis, that is to say that we must see the person and not the diagnosis they have. This idea is basically human; we are all humans after all, and should not be considered as objects of care. Tom Kitwood discovered that all patients, residents, service users and clients who are treated as persons behave like persons to a greater degree than those who are treated as care objects. This means that the way in which the staff care for persons with dementia is of vital importance to the development of their illness.

Kitwood describes how care that fulfils five basic psychological needs has the result that a person can better overcome his illness and thereby maintain a higher level of function for a longer period of time. The five basic needs are:

1. *Comfort.* That the person receives comfort in the form of tenderness, closeness, soothing of anxiety and sorrow, reassurance and a feeling of security that comes from having a fellow human being nearby. The staff must be able to keep things together when they are in danger of falling apart. When the person loses

his self-control we must not lose ours; instead we must support the person in regaining control.

2. *Attachment.* That the person can connect to the staff so that he feels sure of being acknowledged, regardless of his chaos. 'They still like me, even if I have a bad day.' We start from the person's own perception of events and acknowledge it.

3. *Inclusion.* That the person feels that he is part of the fellowship and part of a bigger context, where the feeling is based on the assumption that the group would be worse off if he were not part of it.

4. *Occupation.* That the person has a meaningful occupation which builds on his skills and his life history, and that he is included in the process of life and routine activities.

5. *Identity.* That the person has an identity, knows who he is and can 'tell' his life story. The right to be seen and heard, and to be taken seriously.

Conversely, there is also care that is malignant in nature, that hastens the progression of disease in a person, and that often leads to behaviour that challenges. Tom Kitwood has identified 17 different examples of this and each of these can vary in degree of seriousness. He calls this 'malignant social psychology'. This is about care that is not based on a person's identity, resources and ability to act as an independent and social human being. It is when staff members use methods such as:

- *Intimidation.* It could be threatening to tell the person's spouse that he is not eating.

- *Withholding.* Not giving the person the attention he is asking for.

- *Outpacing.* For example, feeding the person so quickly that he can't keep up (he doesn't have time to swallow or he doesn't feel ready for the next mouthful).

- *Infantilisation.* Treating the person like a child through tone of voice, demands and maybe even friendliness.

- *Labelling.* Calling the person a screamer, stripper or the like. This can also be how we use words such as dementia to create a possibly over-simplified picture of the person.

- *Disparagement.* Telling the person that he is incompetent, worthless, or suchlike.

- *Accusation.* Accusing the person of having done something he shouldn't, or of not having done something he should have done.

- *Treachery.* For example, saying that if the person doesn't do the right thing, we're going to tell the department supervisor.

- *Invalidation.* Discounting the person's experiences. For example, saying that the person can't be hungry since he has just eaten.

- *Disempowerment.* Not allowing the person to use the skills and abilities he has. For example, being too busy to let the person eat at their own speed.

- *Imposition.* Forcing the person to do something or taking away his freedom of choice.

- *Disruption.* Confusing the person in order to get him to do what we want. For example, being so quick to get the person into the shower that he has no opportunity to participate at his own speed.

- *Objectification.* Treating the person as an object. For example, making the bed without speaking to the person while doing so.

- *Stigmatisation.* Treating the person as if he wasn't human and so not in need of consideration.

- *Ignoring.* Speaking over the head of the person one is working with. Unfortunately this happens often, and we need to be aware of it.

- *Banishment.* Sending the person to his room or just actively ignoring him.

- *Mockery.* Making fun of the person, either in his presence or in the staffroom.

But Tom Kitwood is not the only one who describes how staff should or should not behave in relation to the people they work with in older care. Professor Dawn Brooker (2007) built further on Kitwood's work after his all-too-early death, and gives suggestions for alternative ways of working. She has described 17 things to think of for a positive interaction:

- *Warmth.* To show that one really cares about the person one is working with.

- *Holding.* To create a warm and secure everyday life.

- *Relaxed pace.* To work so that the person is able to keep up.

- *Respect.* To treat the person as a worthy citizen and to acknowledge his history and what he has accomplished in life.

- *Acceptance.* To accept the person as he is, from a positive point of departure.

- *Celebration.* To rejoice with the person over his everyday successes.

- *Acknowledgement.* To support the person in his individuality and acknowledge his worth as a person.

- *Genuineness.* To be open about the person's reality without discounting his perception of things. It helps the person to stick to the reality he keeps forgetting.

- *Validation.* To affirm the person's perception of things.

- *Empowerment.* To give the person the possibility of succeeding, and ideally also the support to do so.

- *Facilitation.* To constantly evaluate the need for support and adjust accordingly. One should create the possibility for the person to do as much as possible for himself but, at the same time, always be ready to provide support when it is needed.

- *Enabling.* To encourage the person to choose to do things himself.

- *Collaboration.* To treat the person as an equal by asking the person's advice on how we are to cooperate.

- *Recognition.* To remember what the person likes and dislikes. To know and acknowledge his habits and generally to see him as an individual person.

- *Inclusion.* To work so that the person feels he is part of the fellowship.

- *Belonging.* To create a feeling of belonging in the person and that he belongs together with us as people.

- *Fun.* To make sure that life is full of humour and fun and jokes. This is something we all need.

REFERENCE

Brooker, D. (2007) *Person Centered Dementia Care: Making Service Better*. London: Jessica Kingsley Publishers.

Study Materials

Here are some suggestions for how to structure discussions about the book that you and your colleagues can work from. As a suggestion, you can spend fifteen minutes to half an hour at every staff meeting and gradually work your way through the book.

Enjoy!

PART 1

1 Always identify the one with the problem
Many of the forms of behaviour that challenges we experience in people with dementia are a problem only for us. It is not rare that they themselves see what we consider behaviour that challenges as solutions.

Discuss

- Think of some examples of situations in which you can see that behaviour that challenges actually wasn't a problem for the resident, but only for you as staff.

- Can you remember whether any of these situations led to an escalation of conflict, where you and the person with dementia perceived the situation differently?

2 People behave well if they can

'People behave well if they can' is one of many possible ways of expressing Ross W. Greene's phrase 'Kids do well if they can'. I think it is the formulation with the most power. It is easy to ask too much of a person with dementia, to demand too much of his abilities. The following list of skills that we often ask too much of is our own:

- the ability to calculate cause and effect in complex situations
- the ability to plan and perform activities
- the ability to remember while thinking
- the ability to control impulses
- endurance
- flexibility
- social skills
- sensitivity to stress
- the ability to say 'yes'
- the ability to calm down and remain calm
- the ability to let oneself be urged into a specific behaviour by things with a summoning nature.

Discuss

- Which skills have you expected too much of? Think of some situations for each skill.

- In addition, identify some situations where things have gone badly and in which you can identify the expectations you had that were too high.

- How can you avoid similar situations in the future and instead adjust yourselves so that the residents you work with can live up to expectations?

- Do you think it is enough that you focus on changing expectations, or is it the everyday structure, schedule or physical framework that needs to be changed?

3 People always do what makes sense

We humans are greatly affected by the situations we are a part of, and we usually do what feels right in each situation without really thinking very much about what we are doing. It is the same for people with dementia. The problem is that they may be perceiving the world differently from us and so they act differently to what we expect.

Discuss

- Think about situations in which you truly can understand why the resident did as he did in a particular situation.

- Also identify situations from your own life when perhaps you didn't do what was expected of you by those around you, but in which you did what you did because it was the most understandable choice. Was your behaviour in those situations the best after all, in the long run?

4 Those who take responsibility can make a difference

When we have used a poor method, we often try to get rid of our responsibility. For example by placing it on the relatives instead (it is their fault that we don't succeed in our work), or on colleagues (if they only worked in the same way as we do, things would be better), or the resident (he is stubborn, irritating or something similar), or by discussing whether the person really should be living somewhere else.

Discuss

- Think of situations in which you as staff have tried to get rid of your responsibility:

  - ▸ Do you talk more about the behaviour of certain residents than of others?

  - ▸ Are some of the older people constantly referred to using words like 'stubborn'?

  - ▸ Do you discuss among yourselves whether certain residents should be living somewhere else?

5 People with dementia no longer learn

It is easy to forget that people with dementia no longer learn. To then continue to reprimand them, use consequences, or the like will of course have no effect.

Discuss

- Think of situations that you have managed on the assumption that people with dementia can learn, or learn by failure. What does this assumption mean in your everyday work?

6 You need self-control to cooperate with others
This principle is best discussed together with the next one.

7 Everyone does what they can
to maintain self-control
All humans try to maintain self-control in order to be able to interact with their environment. This applies also to people with dementia. But they may need stronger strategies to maintain their self-control, such as refusing, lying, retreating, or using threats or insults.

Discuss

- Identify situations where what you perceive as behaviour that challenges by the person with dementia is actually a strategy for maintaining self-control. What implications does this insight have for your work in the future?

8 Affect is contagious
We humans feel other people's emotions. People with dementia do so rather more than the rest of us, because they don't know who has the feeling in the first place. This places high demands on the way in which we handle our emotions.

Discuss

- Think of situations in which your affect is transmitted to the residents. It could be anger or unease (stress), but also joy and enthusiasm.

- And even more interesting, see if you can think of situations where the affect of the residents infected you to the point where you lost your overview of the situation and your ability to keep it together.

- Can you come up with possible strategies for minimising the risk of this happening?

9 Conflicts consist of solutions *and* Failures require an action plan

A conflict most often begins by one person having a problem that needs to be solved. But he might solve it in a way that leads to a problem for someone else, which that person in turn must solve. Maybe in a way that leads to a problem for the first person. And so the conflict has begun.

Discuss

- Identify situations where conflicts between you and the residents have had the structure described by this principle. Preferably both situations where you won and situations where you lost.

- Try also to think of situations where people with dementia have had conflicts of this type among themselves.

- How could you have intervened in these situations? Try to think practically based on the situations you have identified.

10 Pedagogy and care involve making the right demands in a way that works

Our work often involves making necessary demands of people with dementia that they would no longer demand of themselves. The demands must therefore be made in such a way that the person with dementia will want to follow them.

Discuss

- Which methods do you use in everyday life to get people with dementia to say 'yes'? Use the bullet list pages 93–95 as a starting point, but also look for methods of your own that we haven't thought of.

- Which distractions do you use? It could be useful to talk about a specific resident in your department and write down the distractions each of you uses, so that you can share them with each other.

11 To lead is to cooperate
Authority is something you receive from others, not something you take.

Discuss

- What do you do to get people with dementia to give you authority? Feel free to share concrete details of the strategies you use.

PART 2

12 We work in a garage
Here it would be a good idea to go back to the principle of responsibility (see Chapter 4).

Discuss

- How does the metaphor of a garage fit in with your work situation? Do you work in a garage or do you have a tendency to:

  ▸ lay the responsibility on the relatives?

▸ lay the blame for the resident's failings on the fact that he doesn't want to cooperate?

▸ think that the resident isn't doing his best in the situation?

▸ use methods that you are comfortable with even though you know that the resident needs other methods?

17 Always exclude the possibility that it could be somatic
Discuss

- Identify situations where it became clear that there was a somatic cause behind a resident's behavioural changes.

- Did you ask the right questions with regard to the changes? Did you use the two rules described in the chapter?

  ▸ If there have been changes in a resident's condition during the past few days or weeks, it is not due to the dementia but due to something somatic.

  ▸ Psychotropic drugs have no effect on dementia symptoms; instead they have a strong sedative effect on the brain and tend to accumulate in the body.

- How can you make sure that you always exclude the possibility that the resident is suffering from something somatic before you move on to pedagogical interventions?

Wishing you the greatest pleasure in your fascinating work!
Bo, Charlotte and Iben

References

In this section you can find references to the thoughts and methods presented in the book, chapter by chapter. We might repeat ourselves along the way, but only to make the connection between the principles more evident.

Introduction
The part on person-centred care is based on:

Kitwood, T. (1997) *Dementia Reconsidered: The Person Comes First.* Maidenhead: Open University Press.

Brooker, D. (2007). *Person Centered Dementia Care: Making Service Better.* London: Jessica Kingsley Publishers

Facts on dementia are from:

David, A.S., Fleminger S., Kopelman, M.D., Lovestone, S., Mellers, J.D.C., and Lishman, W.A. (2009) *Organic Psychiatry: A Textbook of Neuropsychiatry.* Oxford: Blackwell Science.

PART 1

1 Always identify the one with the problem

This chapter is based on thinking introduced by Andrew McDonnell in his book:

> McDonnell, A. (2010) *Managing Aggressive Behavior in Care Settings.* London: Wiley.

It is also the basis of:

> Elvén, B.H. (2010) *No Fighting, No Biting, No Screaming: How to Make Behaving Positively Possible for People with Autism and Other Developmental Disabilities.* London: Jessica Kingsley Publishers.

2 People behave well if they can

Ross W. Greene's work is on children, but we believe that it is a global principle. He first formulated the principle in his book:

> Greene, R.W. (2014) *The Explosive Child: A New Approach for Understanding and Parenting Easily Frustrated, Chronically Inflexible Children.* London: Harper Paperbacks.

If you want to learn more on executive function you can read:

> Gazzaniga, M.S., Ivry, R.B., and Mangun, G.R. (2013) *Cognitive Neuroscience.* New York: Norton.

Greene keeps an updated reference list on his website: www. livesinthebalance.org.

The list of skills we often place high demands on is our own. But there is a lot to read on every skill:

The ability to calculate cause and effect in complex situations
You can find a lot of both research and theory on the subject of *central coherence*, for example:

Happé, F. (2013) 'Weak Central Coherence.' In F.R. Volkmar (ed.) *Encyclopedia of Autism Spectrum Disorders.* New York: Springer.

The ability to structure, plan and carry out activities

Gazzaniga, M.S., Ivry, R.B., and Mangun, G.R. (2013) *Cognitive Neuroscience.* New York: Norton.

The ability to remember while thinking

Baddeley, A. (2007) *Working Memory, Thought, and Action* (Oxford Psychology Series). Oxford: Oxford University Press.

The ability to restrain impulses

Gazzaniga, M.S., Ivry, R.B., and Mangun, G.R. (2013) *Cognitive Neuroscience.* New York: Norton.

Stamina
A great popular science article:

Lehrer, J. (2009) 'Don't: The secret of self-control.' *The New Yorker*, May 18. www.newyorker.com/reporting /2009/05 /18/090518fa_fact_lehrer.

The ability to be flexible
An older defining article:

Scott, W.A. (1962) 'Cognitive complexity and cognitive flexibility.' *American Sociological Association 25*, 405–414.

Social abilities

Frith, U. (2003) *Autism: Explaining the Enigma.* London: Wiley.

Resilience to stress
If you really want to understand stress I recommend that you read Chapter 4 in:

Elvén, B.H. (2010) *No Fighting, No Biting, No Screaming: How to Make Behaving Positively Possible for People with Autism and Other Developmental Disabilities.* London: Jessica Kingsley Publishers.

The ability to say 'yes'

DiStefano, C., Morgan, G.B., and Motl, R.W. (2012) 'An examination of personality characteristics related to acquiescence.' *Journal of Applied Measurement 13*, 1, 41–56.

The ability to calm down or to remain calm

Diekhof, E.K., Geier, K., Falkai, P., and Gruber, O. (2011) 'Fear is only as deep as the mind allows. A coordinate-based meta-analysis of neuroimaging studies on the regulation of negative affect.' *Neuroimage 58*, 1, 275–285.

Sjöwall, D., Roth, L., Lindqvist, S., and Thorell, L.B. (2013) 'Multiple deficits in ADHD: executive dysfunction, delay aversion, reaction time variability, and emotional deficits.' *Journal of Child Psychology and Psychiatry 54*, 6, 619–627.

3 People always do what makes sense

You can read about how physical environments affect behaviour in:

Norman, D. (1988) *The Psychology of Everyday Things.* New York: Basic Books.

On structure as a tool:

Kabot, S., and Reeve, C. (2012) *Building Independence: How to Create and Use Structured Work Systems.* USA: Autism Asperger Publishing Co.

On making sense by the well known:

Kitwood, T. (1997) *Dementia Reconsidered: The Person Comes First.* Maidenhead: Open University Press.

4 Those who take responsibility can make a difference

The quote is adapted from:

Weiner, B. (1995) *Judgments of Responsibility: A Foundation for a Theory of Social Conduct.* New York: Guilford Press.

Dave Dagnan's work:

Dagnan, D., and Cairns, M. (2005) 'Staff judgements of responsibility for the challenging behaviour of adults with intellectual disabilities.' *Journal of Intellectual Disability Research 49,* 1, 95–101.

In this chapter we write about punishment. Maybe we need to clarify that we use the term punishment as it is used by most people. We don't use it as it is used in behaviouristic theory. If you want to read more on the negative effects of punishment you can read:

Gershoff, E.T. (2002) 'Corporal punishment by parents and associated child behaviors and experiences: a meta-analytic and theoretical review.' *Psychological Bulletin 128*, 4, 539–579.

Shutters, S.T. (2013) 'Collective action and the detrimental side of punishment.' *Evolutionary Psychology 11*, 2, 327–346.

Sigsgaard, E. (2005) *Scolding: Why It Hurts More Than It Helps.* New York: Teachers College Press.

On legitimising effects:

Gneezy, U., and Rustichini, A. (2000) 'A fine is a price.' *The Journal of Legal Studies 29*, 1, 1–17.

On why we punish even if it doesn't work:

de Quervain, D.J.F., Fischbacher, U., Treyer, V., Schellhammer M., *et al.* (2004) 'The neural basis of altruistic punishment.' *Science 305*, 1254–1258.

Boyd, R., Gintis, H., Bowles, S., and Richerson, P.J. (2003) 'The evolution of altruistic punishment.' *Proceedings of the National Academy of Science USA 100*, 6, 3531–3535.

5 People with dementia no longer learn

The chapter is based on the article:

van Duijvenvoorde, A.C.K., Zanolie, K., Rombouts, S.A.R.B., Raijmakers, M.E.J., and Crone, E.A. (2008) 'Evaluating the negative or valuing the positive? Neural mechanisms supporting feedback-based learning across development.' *The Journal of Neuroscience 28*, 38, 9495–9503.

6 You need self-control to cooperate with others

Kaplan and Wheeler's original article:

Kaplan, S.G., and Wheeler, E.G. (1983) 'Survival skills for working with potentially violent clients.' *Social Casework 64*, 339–345.

Our model was first published in:

Elvén, B.H. (2010) *No Fighting, No Biting, No Screaming: How to Make Behaving Positively Possible for People with Autism and Other Developmental Disabilities.* London: Jessica Kingsley Publishers.

Other selected readings:

Diekhof, E.K., Geier, K., Falkai, P., and Gruber, O. (2011) 'Fear is only as deep as the mind allows. A coordinate-based meta-analysis of neuroimaging studies on the regulation of negative affect.' *Neuroimage 58*, 1, 275–285.

Sjöwall, D., Roth, L., Lindqvist, S., and Thorell, L.B. (2013) 'Multiple deficits in ADHD: executive dysfunction, delay aversion, reaction time variability, and emotional deficits.' *Journal of Child Psychology and Psychiatry 54*, 6, 619–627.

7 Everyone does what they can to maintain self-control

Elvén, B.H. (2010) *No Fighting, No Biting, No Screaming: How to Make Behaving Positively Possible for People with Autism and Other Developmental Disabilities.* London: Jessica Kingsley Publishers.

A great popular science article on lying:

Bronson, P. (2008) 'Learning to lie.' *New York Magazine.* http://nymag.com/news/features/43893.

8 Affect is contagious

The concept of affect contagion comes from:

Tomkins, S. (1962) *Affect, Imagery, Consciousness: Volume I.* London: Tavistock.

Tomkins, S. (1963) *Affect, Imagery, Consciousness: Volume II, The Negative Affects.* New York: Springer.

Tomkins, S. (1991) *Affect, Imagery, Consciousness: Volume III. The Negative Affects: Anger and Fear.* New York: Springer.

Scientific basis:

Hatfield, E., Cacioppo, J.T., and Rapson, R.L. (1993) 'Emotional contagion.' *Current Directions in Psychological Science 2*, 3, 96–99.

A great popular book on the subject is:

Nathanson, D.L. (1992) *Shame and Pride: Affect, Sex, and the Birth of the Self.* New York: Norton.

The mirror neuron research:

Rizzolatti, G., and Craighero, L. (2004) 'The mirror-neuron system.' *Annual Review of Neuroscience 27*, 169–192.

The Daniel Stern quote is from a talk he gave at the conference *Meeting of Minds* in Herning, Denmark, in 2007.

The strategies for lowering the affect are from the low-arousal approach. You can read more on that in:

Elvén, B.H. (2010) *No Fighting, No Biting, No Screaming: How to Make Behaving Positively Possible for People with Autism and Other Developmental Disabilities.* London: Jessica Kingsley Publishers.

McDonnell, A. (2010) *Managing Aggressive Behavior in Care Settings.* London: Wiley.

9 Conflicts consist of solutions *and* Failures require an action plan

Scientific documentation on restraint-related deaths:

Nunno, M.A., Holden, M.J., and Tollar, A. (2006) 'Learning from tragedy: a survey of child and adolescent restraint fatalities.' *Child Abuse & Neglect 30*, 1333–1342.

Aiken, F., Duxbury, J., Dale, C., and Harbison, I. (2011) *Review of the Medical Theories and Research Relating to Restraint Related Deaths.* Lancaster: Caring Solutions (UK), University of Central Lancashire.

Lieberman, J.L., Dodd, C.J., Moynihan, D.P., Domenici, P.V., *et al.* (1999) *Improper Restraint or Seclusion Use Places People at Risk.* United States General Accounting Office, Report to Congressional Requesters.

Paterson, B., Bradley, P., Stark, C., Saddler, D., Leadbetter, D., and Allen, D. (2003) 'Deaths associated with restraint use in health and social care in the UK. The results of a preliminary survey.' *Journal of Psychiatric and Mental Health Nursing 10*, 3–15.

On how a decrease in restraints decreases injuries:

Holstead, J., Lamond, D., Dalton, J., Horne, A., and Crick, R. (2010) 'Restraint reduction in children's residential facilities: implementation at damar services.' *Residential Treatment for Children & Youth 27*, 1–13.

10 Pedagogy and care involve making the right demands in a way that works

Martha Nussbaum's thoughts on autonomy:

Nussbaum, M.C. (2007) *Frontiers of Justice: Disability, Nationality, Species Membership* (The Tanner Lectures on Human Values). Boston: Harvard University Press.

On violence towards the one who sets limits:

Bjørkly, S. (1999) 'A ten-year prospective study of aggression in a special secure unit for dangerous patients.' *Scandinavian Journal of Psychology 40*, 1, 57–63.

On diversion:

Smith, R.E. (1973) 'The use of humor in the counterconditioning of anger responses: a case study.' *Behavior Therapy 4*, 4, 576–580.

McDonnell, A. (2010) *Managing Aggressive Behavior in Care Settings.* London: Wiley.

Elvén, B.H. (2010) *No Fighting, No Biting, No Screaming: How to Make Behaving Positively Possible for People with Autism and Other Developmental Disabilities.* London: Jessica Kingsley Publishers.

On how to get a 'yes':

> Elvén, B.H. (2010) *No Fighting, No Biting, No Screaming: How to Make Behaving Positively Possible for People with Autism and Other Developmental Disabilities.* London: Jessica Kingsley Publishers.

11 To lead is to cooperate

Hobbes' thoughts on power are from:

> Hobbes, T. (1651/1982) *Leviathan.* London: Penguin Classics.

Rawls' thoughts are from:

> Rawls, J. (1971) *A Theory of Justice.* Cambridge, MA: Belknap Press of Harvard University Press.

Martha Nussbaum's thoughts on autonomy:

> Nussbaum, M.C. (2007) *Frontiers of Justice: Disability, Nationality, Species Membership* (The Tanner Lectures on Human Values). Boston: Harvard University Press.

PART 2

The model builds on:

> Kaplan, S.G., and Wheeler, E.G. (1983) 'Survival skills for working with potentially violent clients.' *Social Casework 64*, 339–345.

> Whitaker, P. (2001) *Challenging Behaviour and Autism: Making Sense, Making Progress.* London: National Autistic Society.

The model was first published in:

Elvén, B.H. (2010) *No Fighting, No Biting, No Screaming: How to Make Behaving Positively Possible for People with Autism and Other Developmental Disabilities.* London: Jessica Kingsley Publishers.

The plans are based on a Swedish project:

Björne, P., Andresson, I., Björne, M., Olsson, M., and Pagmert, S. (2012) *Utmanande Beteenden, Utmanande Verksamheter.* Malmö: Stadskontoret.

You can read more on physical interventions in:

McDonnell, A. (2010) *Managing Aggressive Behavior in Care Settings.* London: Wiley.